# The Sneeze-Free Cat Owner

Diane Morgan

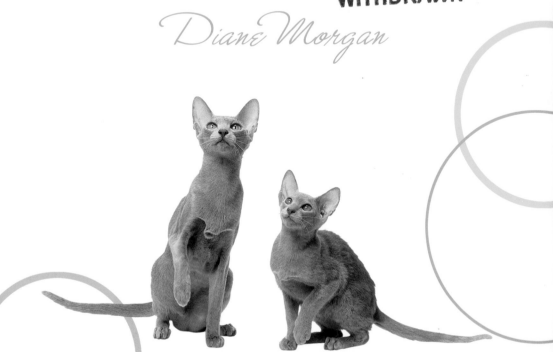

*The Sneeze-Free Cat Owner*
Diane Morgan

Project Team
Editor: Mary E. Grangeia
Copy Editor: Stephanie Fornino
Designer: Stephanie Krautheim

T.F.H. Publications
President/CEO: Glen S. Axelrod
Executive Vice President: Mark E. Johnson
Publisher: Christopher T. Reggio
Production Manager: Kathy Bontz

T.F.H. Publications, Inc.
One TFH Plaza
Third and Union Avenues
Neptune City, NJ 07753

Printed and bound in China

07 08 09 10 11 1 3 5 7 9 8 6 4 2

Library of Congress Cataloging-in-Publication Data
Morgan, Diane, 1947-
  The sneeze-free cat owner / Diane Morgan.
     p. cm.
  Includes index.
  ISBN 978-0-7938-0605-8 (alk. paper)
  1. Cats. 2. Cat breeds. 3. Cats--Selection. 4. Allergens--Control. 5. Allergy. I. Title.
SF442.M66 2007
636.8--dc22
                                        2006039148

This book has been published with the intent to provide accurate and authoritative information in regard to the subject matter within. While every precaution has been taken in preparation of this book, the author and publisher expressly disclaim responsibility for any errors, omissions, or adverse effects arising from the use or application of the information contained herein. The techniques and suggestions are used at the reader's discretion and are not to be considered a substitute for veterinary care. If you suspect a medical problem consult your veterinarian.

*The Leader In Responsible Animal Care For Over 50 Years!*™
www.tfh.com

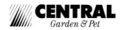

# Chapters

contents . . . . . . ○○○○○

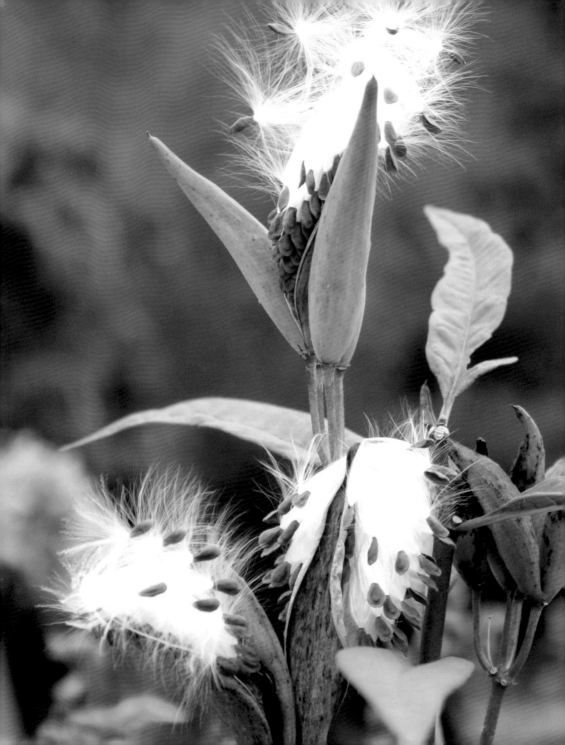

# *Welcome to*
# ALLERGY WORLD

I said something which gave you to think I hated cats. But gad, sir, I am one of the most fanatical cat lovers in the business. If you hate them, I may learn to hate you. If your allergies hate them, I will tolerate the situation to the best of my ability.

—Raymond Chandler (1888-1959) in a letter to publisher Hamish Hamilton, Jan. 26, 1950

# Cats

are possibly the most beautiful, graceful, and elegant of all earth's creatures. They are easy to care for, simple to housetrain, and provide their owners with regular, if moderate, affection. They don't need to be taken for walks, don't require "kitten socialization classes," and almost never attack the letter carrier. They even keep themselves sparkling clean. Cats are, in so many ways, the ideal pet. What a shame, then, that so many people are allergic to them.

According to the Asthma and Allergy Foundation of America (AAFA), more than 50 million Americans suffer from allergies. Of those, millions suffer from some sort of pet allergy. And with 70 percent of families owning a cat or dog, those statistics are certainly nothing to sneeze at! In fact, allergies are the most widespread chronic condition on the planet.

Cats aren't the only allergy-causing creatures, of course. In fact, a 2003 study suggested that more people are actually allergic to their dogs. Many can also be allergic to rabbits, birds, horses, guinea pigs, mice, and gerbils. Laboratory and zoo workers have been found to be allergic to monkeys, tigers, and lions. People with mold allergies can develop allergy symptoms from bird droppings and the accumulation of mold in cages. Poorly kept fish tanks can develop mold also, which leads some to believe that they are allergic to their fish.

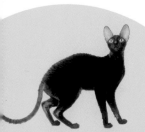

Most people who are allergic to cats are allergic to other things as well. In addition, the more "other things" one is allergic to, the worse the symptoms of the allergy become.

As it turns out, between 2 and 15 percent of the world's population is allergic to cats, and four out of every five people who are allergic to animals are allergic to cats. About a third of these sufferers are living with one. Even people who don't live with cats can be affected. Cat allergens have been found in almost one-third of noncat owners' homes and on the clothing of coworkers who don't own any animals. And while many owners tough it out, the sad fact is that a great many cats given up to shelters are there because their humans are allergic to them.

Once upon a time it was standard operating procedure for physicians to blithely tell their patients to "find the cat another home." But that's not an option for most people nowadays. Our cats are no longer disposable barnyard hunters but instead cherished members of the family. We recognize them as living beings with real value that extends beyond any usefulness they may have as killers of mice. As we have so tragically seen in the aftermath of numerous natural disasters, many people would not abandon

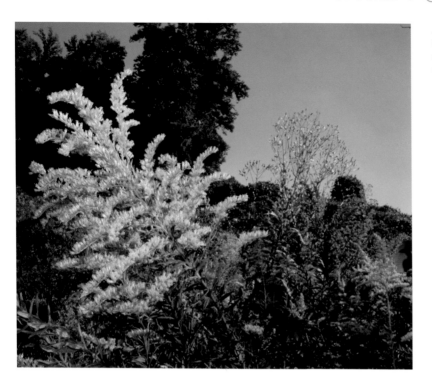

*Allergies are one of the most widespread chronic conditions throughout the world.*

their faithful pets even in the face of life-threatening events, much less give them away because of some sneezing. Others work around animals as part of their jobs; still more need the help of an assistance pet. And no one can underestimate their benefit to the elderly and lonely.

Yet there's no doubt that allergies can make people sick and miserable. All is not lost, however. This is the 21st century. Allergies can be managed, if not actually cured. The contemporary cat owner has the ways and means to keep her cat and kick the cough. Despite what an old-fashioned doctor may claim, Fluffy does not have to live in the barn or go to the shelter, although as we shall see, you may have to lock her out of the bedroom.

Besides, it's not even realistic to think that "getting rid" of an animal will "get rid" of allergies—not unless you move to a pet-free planet or at least live in a bubble. And most homes are not bubbles; pet allergens can hang around in carpets and on furniture for a long time. A study from the National Institute for Environmental Health Sciences makes this clear. Researchers investigated 831 homes across the entire country. All types of

Scientists have found that male cats produce more allergenic sebaceous secretions than females. (It's a function of testosterone.) Neutered cats therefore produce fewer allergens than intact ones. It's always nice to find yet another good reason to neuter your cat.

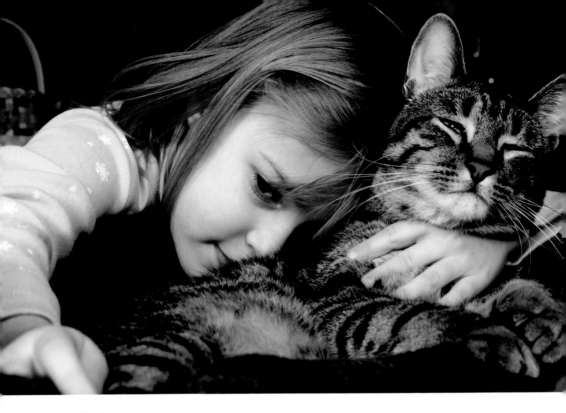

*Pets of all kinds can cause allergic responses, which for some people can result in other health problems as well.*

housing were tested in rural as well as urban areas. Every one of them contained pet allergens, including those homes that had no resident pet. Nine percent of the *catless* homes contained enough allergens to provoke an asthma attack in anyone allergic to felines.

Pets of all kinds can cause allergic responses, which for some folks, can result in other health problems as well. Most symptoms are rather mild. We might cough or sneeze. We might itch. Our eyes might turn red or tear up. Our noses may run. Reactions will vary from one individual to the next.

Allergies manifest themselves in several different ways: sneezing and a runny or stuffy nose (allergic rhinitis); sinusitis (inflammation of the nasal cavity); ear infections; conjunctivitis (inflammation of the lining of the eye); dermatitis (inflammation of the skin); itching; or hives. Some people have more serious reactions, including asthma. In rare cases (usually due to some injected allergen), an allergy can cause a deadly reaction called anaphylaxis. Thankfully, cat allergens don't produce this reaction, although insect sting venom, shellfish, and peanuts can. To make things worse, an allergy can sometimes seem to appear overnight, although in actual fact it was years in the making. So what causes it?

In the past, it was commonly believed that animal hair caused allergies, but with pets, the villainous substance is not hair at all. While the responsible allergen can definitely be found in a feline's fur, that's not where it originates. Allergies are triggered by special proteins called allergens, which are secreted by oil glands in the skin and shed with dander. Allergenic proteins are also abundant in saliva, which indeed clings to hair. Still more allergens can be found in urine, feces, serum, mucus, dander, and hair roots.

Even though hair is made from protein, it's a harmless protein that almost no one is allergic to. With cats, the bad protein actually comes from their saliva in the form of a vicious little protein called Fel d1 (short for *Felis domesticus*). When the cat licks herself, she deposits her saliva on her fur, where it coats the dander, then dries, floats merrily away, and enters the nose of the allergy sufferer.

Airborne allergens are the hardest ones to avoid. Cat allergens, for instance, are everywhere. They have even been found in Antarctica, traveling on the wings of the wind—and there are no cats living on the

Contrary to popular belief, it's not a cat's fur that causes allergies; it's the oil-producing glands of the skin that produce proteins called allergens.

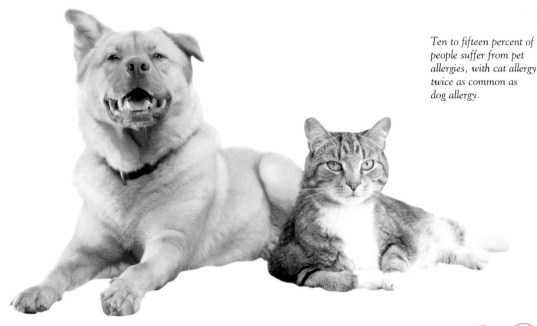

*Ten to fifteen percent of people suffer from pet allergies, with cat allergy twice as common as dog allergy.*

Children under the age of 18 are more likely to suffer from allergies than adults aged 18 to 64.

entire continent. In North America, where there are 73 million domestic cats and another 60 million feral cats, allergens are even more prevalent.

Allergies are here to stay, and many believe that the culprit protein is very sticky and so light that it floats everywhere and clings to everything. Studies have suggested that most allergens are brought into the home by visitors and deposited on sofas, chairs, etc. Whether the visitors themselves owned cats or dogs or had merely captured some allergens sailing by on the wind was not determined. In other words, these sticky little proteins are impossible to escape—although, admittedly, levels are higher in homes that house an indoor pet. Nevertheless, anywhere you sit, you are picking up and depositing pet allergens.

The bottom line is that animal dander, which is nothing more than dead skin cells, is a major contributing factor in causing allergies, and it's produced not only by cats and dogs but by all birds and mammals, including people. If you are not willing to put up with dander but still want a pet, you may want to consider a tarantula, scorpion, or python. However, these pets also have their drawbacks, so your best bet is to learn what you can do to minimize and manage those allergies so that you and your pet can live happily and well.

*Although it's commonly believed that animal hair causes allergies, the culprit is actually an allergenic protein in the cat's saliva that gets deposited on the fur when she licks herself.*

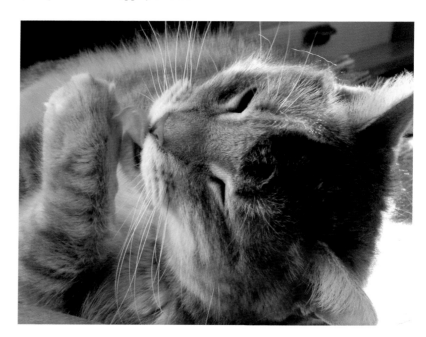

## RECOGNIZING A PET ALLERGY

Some people who are allergic to their own pets have no severe or immediate increase of their symptoms when they are near them. Instead, they suffer from continual low-grade symptoms that clear up only after days or even weeks away from the house.

The most common symptoms related to cat exposure are:

- red, itchy, or swollen eyes
- reddened areas on the skin
- runny nose, nasal congestion, and post-nasal drip
- sneezing
- itchy or stuffed-up ears
- hoarse or itchy throat
- coughing and wheezing
- frequent bronchitis

Animal dander can also cause what is called "perennial allergic rhinitis," the sneezing and runny nose that result from breathing in these airborne particles. Rather oddly, most people with this type of allergy don't have eye inflammation, but they do get nasal congestion that can block the eustachian tubes and cause hearing problems, especially in children. Complications of pet allergy can include chronic sinus headaches and infections, and even asthma.

The trouble begins when the animal dander encounters the mucous membranes of your nose or the bronchial tubes of your throat. Bits of cat dander are very small (2.5 microns or 1/25,000 of an inch). They can stay airborne for hours, even in motionless air. Particularly potent and invisible to the eye, the offending protein can trigger an allergic reaction within minutes. The stuff dries and flakes into tiny particles like aerosol droplets. To give you an idea of what I am talking about here, cat allergen is about ten times *smaller* than pollen or dust particles; it is so small that it easily penetrates the bronchial membranes.

The good news is that about 1 in every 50,000 cats apparently lacks the allergy-provoking protein. More about them (and how you can have one for your very own) later.

Before we discuss the breeds that may be less allergenic, let's explore a little bit about what allergies are, what triggers them, and how they are diagnosed. Finding an allergist who will help you in your fight against pet dander without insisting you "get rid" of your pet is the first step in winning the allergy battle.

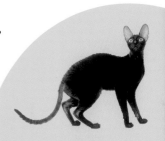

Cat allergies tend to be cumulative and may build up over time. Usually, however, allergies begin in childhood because a child's immune system is much more sensitive than that of an adult.

**Did You Know?**

Cat allergen is about ten times smaller than pollen or dust particles, so it easily irritates your nasal membranes.

## WHAT IS AN ALLERGY?

In simplest terms, an allergy is the result of a misfiring immune system. Normally, the immune system is an excellent thing, keeping us safe from pathological bacteria, viruses, and fungi. But just like the rest of the body, it can make mistakes. An allergic reaction occurs when the immune system gets a little out of whack and ends up attacking its owner instead of the invasive bodies.

It can be hard to distinguish among perennial allergic rhinitis, recurring sinus infections, or polyps inside the nose, especially when someone has all three at the same time.

### Immunology 101

While the finer points of immunology are somewhat obscure, the fundamentals are easy to understand. One way that we repel invaders is to lock them out, which is one of the functions of our skin and even the tiny hairs inside our noses. When the invaders get inside, the body needs to call upon its immune cells for defense.

People with allergies have "hyperactive" immune systems. The first time a potentially allergic person encounters a cat allergen, nothing happens—it seems. But the immune system is actually hard at work. Plasma cells, which are located just under the mucous membranes, begin churning up antibodies to fight the offending protein.

Allergic people tend to make a good deal of a special antibody called immunoglobulin E (IgE). A big protein shaped somewhat like the letter Y,

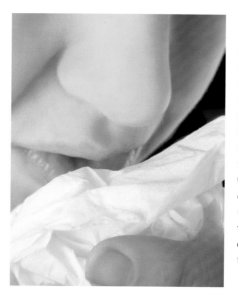

*The most common cat allergy symptoms are sneezing, itchy eyes and throat, and a runny nose.*

it's called the "allergen antibody" because it causes immediate, acute reactions to irritating substances. IgE hooks onto the mast cells and basophils (special cells found in the mucosal tissue of the lungs, skin, and tongue, and the linings of the nose and intestinal tract) that line the nose and bronchial tubes. Called granulocytes, these cells contain powerful substances (yes, called granules) loaded with mighty invader-killing chemicals that are ready to go to work.

Amazingly, the body can tailor its immunoglobulin molecules to fit allergens like a key in a lock. As soon as they come into contact with any invader, the antibodies go into action and you begin to suffer allergy symptoms. And what's more, once they have "introduced themselves," they now just wait around until they meet the allergens again. Your immune system is primed. The next time allergens are breathed in, the antibodies catch hold of them and send out signals for reinforcements, which include other allergy attackers like histamine and heparin (and about 30 others).

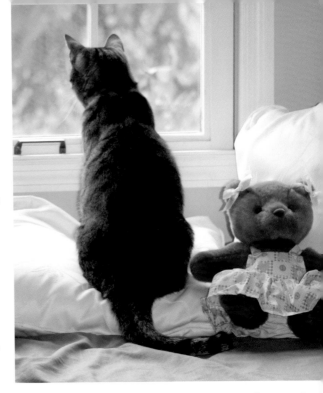

The way these fighting antibodies try to expel invaders is by making you sneeze and snivel. They have no way of knowing, apparently, that cat allergens are not smallpox or worms! (Some people think that the original purpose of IgE was to rid the body of internal parasites.) Several researchers guess that the discomfort associated with these symptoms is nature's way of telling you to stay away from the particular allergen in the future. It is too bad that no one told the allergic immune system that *it* was the problem, not the cat hair or the ragweed. To make things worse, the body can produce different kinds of IgE for different substances, which is why people often develop multiple allergies.

In addition to an immediate reaction, some people may experience a delayed reaction up to several hours later. This occurs with the arrival of still more trooper cells, like eosinophils, neutrophils, and lymphocytes, at the site of the invasion. From the sufferer's point of view, these guys are even worse because they can cause actual tissue damage.

*Because pet allergies tend to build up over time, they may not show up right away. Be sure to spend some time around cats before deciding to bring one home.*

## First Exposure

Interestingly, the first exposure to an allergen doesn't result in symptoms, even for those who later develop an allergy. The first exposure simply encourages antibodies to be produced. With repeated exposure over

**Did You Know?**

Histamine is fondly known by some allergy sufferers as the "allergy bomb."

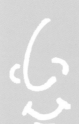

### Antibody Facts

- "Immunoglobulin" and "antibody" are terms that are often used interchangeably.

- Histamines are the most notable but not the only chemicals released by the IgE mast cell combo. Others include prostaglandins, bradykinin, and something called Substance P.

- Besides IgE, human beings make four other kinds of antibodies: IgA, IgD, IgG, and IgM. Luckily, we don't need to talk about them. IgE causes enough trouble all on its own.

- IgE accounts for only about 0.001 percent of the antibody in the blood. It doesn't seem like much, but it obviously is.

If you are considering getting tested, see an ABAI- (American Board of Allergy and Immunology) certified physician for best results. An ABAI doctor has completed a two- to three-year fellowship of specialized study in allergies, in addition to regular medical training.

a period of weeks to years, more and more histamine is released, and that's when symptoms begin.

When we are born, the level of IgE circulating in the bloodstream is very low compared to that of other immunoglobulins. In fact, it's almost nonexistent (although some studies show that higher than normal levels in cord blood and the infant's serum do predict early onset of allergies). In adults, the level of IgE in the system can predict the allergy status of the individual fairly accurately.

Sometimes the term "atopic allergy" is used to refer to the IgE-mediated allergies, such as the cat allergy (Fel d1). However, a person who has an atopic allergy does not seem to be at increased risk for developing an adverse reaction to an *injected* allergen like a vaccination, medication, or insect sting. Atopic allergies are largely inherited. In fact, someone with one allergic parent has almost a 50 percent risk of developing an allergy himself. A person with two allergic parents has a 70 percent risk. So if you're allergic, it's more reasonable to blame your parents than the family cat.

### Identifying the Allergen

Before you blithely assume that your allergy (if it is an allergy) is the cat's fault, get yourself tested. You might be surprised. You could be allergic to mold, dust, or pollen! This isn't really good news because it's even harder to get away from dust than from cats, but at least the Siamese is off the hook. The only definitive way to discover what you are allergic to is by having one of several medical tests.

## Serum-Based Tests

Blood tests to detect allergies are becoming increasingly popular because they are very simple and require little expertise. Unfortunately, these tests can deliver false positives, resulting in treatment being administered for nonexistent allergies.

Serum-based tests work by measuring IgE in the blood. The theory is that if the IgE level is significantly elevated in relation to a suspected allergic substance, you are allergic to that substance. However, even if your IgE level is increased, it doesn't necessarily mean that there is enough of it to cause an allergic reaction. This is how false positives can occur.

## Skin Testing

A blood test can confirm that an allergy is present, but a skin test can actually identify the particular allergy. In fact, there are three different types of skin tests commonly administered.

*Finding an allergist who will help you in your fight against pet dander without insisting you "get rid" of your pet is the first step in winning the allergy battle.*

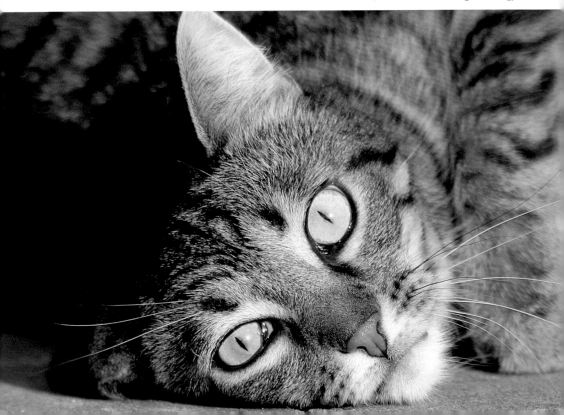

In one kind of skin test, the skin prick/scratch/puncture test, the physician takes dilute solutions of various suspected allergens (pollens, dust, grasses, and animal dander) and scratches them individually into various areas on the skin. If you're allergic to the Fel d1 often present in animal dander, a red swelling called a weal will form at the site within 20 minutes. The advantages of this test are that it is simple, quick, and inexpensive. It can also be used to test any age group, including babies.

In another test, the allergens are injected (usually on the inner forearm). This test is given if the physician suspects an allergy to injected allergens like insect venom. In this test, small markings are placed on the skin in a specific pattern. At each pen mark, a specific substance (potential allergic substance) is injected. Twenty-four to 48 hours later, the skin is examined to determine signs of allergy. Although the test is not 100 percent accurate, most allergies can be determined using this method.

The third test is the skin patch test, which is also considered very accurate and produces few false positives. The suspected allergen is applied to a patch that is placed on the skin. This test is usually given when the physician thinks that the patient may have contact dermatitis from a substance like latex; it's not often given for a suspected allergy to pet dander.

If a skin test cannot be taken for some reason, your physician can perform a radioallergosorbent (RAST) assay, which is equally accurate. A blood sample is taken and sent to a special laboratory to be analyzed to determine how much of a specific kind of IgE antibody is present. RASTs, although safer, are less likely than skin prick tests to pick up sensitivity to allergens and fewer allergenic substances can be tested at once. This test is also more expensive and slower to reveal results.

## Complementary and Alternative Methods to Diagnose Allergies

Just as many practitioners of alternative medicine disagree with conventional Western medicine about how to treat an allergy, they tend to diagnose them differently as well (although the detection methods may look superficially similar). Methods used by some holistic practitioners to detect allergies include the following (in alphabetical order):

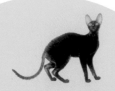

Many tests require that you stop taking medication for allergies sometime prior to getting tested because it can interfere with results. Some of these medications include prescription nonsedating antihistamines such as fexofenadine (Allegra) and cetirizine (Zyrtec), over-the-counter antihistamines (Benadryl, Chlor-Trimeton, and others), tricyclic antidepressants such as amitriptyline and doxepin (Sinequan), and even heartburn medications such as cimetidine (Tagamet) and ranitidine (Zantac).

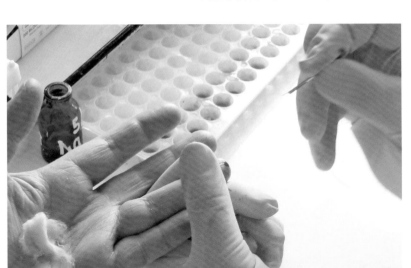

*Before you assume that your allergy is the cat's fault, get yourself tested. You might be surprised to discover you're allergic to mold, dust, or pollen.*

**Antigen Leukocyte Cellular Antibody Test (ALCAT).** In this test, the practitioner draws blood samples and then exposes them to 150 to 200 different extracts of foods, drugs, chemicals, pollens, molds, and animal dander. A computer analyzes changes in leukocytes, a type of blood cell. If the blood cells flatten, fragment, or disintegrate in response to an extract, an allergy to that substance is probably present.

**Applied Kinesiology Testing.** Using this method, the practitioner asks the patient to hold a glass vial containing a suspected allergen in one hand while he bends his opposite arm to measure muscle strength. A decrease in strength is considered a sign of allergy.

**Cytotoxic Testing.** This test is similar to the ALCAT. The practitioner draws samples of blood and exposes them to different extracts. The difference is that instead of results being determined by a computer, a technician actually looks through a microscope for evidence of cellular changes that might indicate allergy. However, according to the American Academy of Allergy, Asthma, and Immunology (AAAAI), a number of clinical trials have found these tests completely ineffective at diagnosing allergies. Such testing is therefore not recommended.

**Provocation-Neutralization Testing.** In this test, a practitioner places drops of suspected allergens under the tongue (sublingual testing) or injects them under the skin. The dose is gradually increased until one is found

There's a condition called vasomotor rhinitis that causes allergy-like symptoms but has nothing to do with allergies.

*While allergies can't be cured, they can usually be controlled—even if you have a cat.*

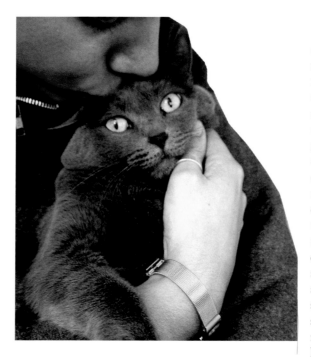

Up to 50 percent of people who are allergic to cats will not have any immediate symptoms. Allergies may not appear until you've been exposed continuously over a period of time; it can take several days to three years for the body to build up enough antibodies to respond. Others find that their symptoms lessen after a period of exposure!

(the provocation dose) that causes any symptom that may be interpreted as an allergic reaction. Then the dose is gradually decreased until one is found (the neutralization dose) that relieves the symptom. This method could be dangerous. If you are extremely allergic to a substance, sublingual testing might trigger a life-threatening anaphylactic reaction. This approach, by the way, is not the same as the traditional desensitization injections given by medical allergy specialists. This test is unproven and not recommended by the AAAAI.

[None of these methodologies have been proven to actually diagnose allergies.]

## HYPOALLERGENIC BREEDS?

In a word, maybe. The prefix "hypo" means "low" or "less than." A hypoallergenic cat would be one who produces fewer allergens than a "regular" cat. However, there are no scientific or legal definitions of this word.

Unfortunately, there seems to be no such thing (at present) as a true hypoallergenic cat breed. In fact, there is no scientific data whatsoever to support the claim that one breed is less allergic than another. In reality, the biggest difference in allergen production is due to the sexual status of the cat: Unneutered males produce by far the highest number of allergens. Even this is a highly individual matter, though—one particular male may be more allergenic than another.

To make things even more confusing, there is considerable allergen variation among different individual cats of the same breed and even at differing times in the same cat, with kittens producing less allergens than adults. This is a sad fact of life. You play with an adoptable kitten, decide you're not allergic after all, and then several months later, the sneezes start. It's not in your head. Kittens have soft, supple skin and don't produce allergens in the same numbers as grown cats do. Even cat-allergic persons can often handle a kitten without suffering a reaction. As the kitten grows, the skin toughens and the sebaceous glands begin producing more sebum, a kind of oil. Sebum may be annoying and allergenic to us, but cats need it to keep their coats in order.

*Unfortunately, hypoallergenic doesn't mean nonallergenic.* The Cornish Rex cat is a particular example of a breed that is often acquired because breeders tout it as being hypoallergenic. Yet it has been estimated that 25 percent of cats sold under this rubric are eventually given up to shelters, simply because they didn't live up to their advanced billing. It does seem to be true that about 10 percent of people allergic to cats tolerate Rex breeds, possibly because they tend to shed less. Those aren't good enough odds to take a gamble on, though.

Another hypoallergenic breed is the Devon. This breed has fewer guard hairs than most. They are low shedders and so release less dander. The coat texture may also help to slough off allergenic proteins from the saliva. The hairless Sphynx may also fall into the "less allergenic" category. But we'll talk about these breeds and more in Chapter 4.

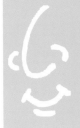

## Different Cats, Different Symptoms

During the annual meeting of the American College of Asthma, Allergy, and Immunology (ACAAI) in Seattle in 2000, an interesting study was presented. It found that people who owned dark-colored cats were two to four times more likely to experience moderate or severe allergic symptoms than people with no cats or with light-colored cats. Even stranger, there was no statistical difference in symptoms between those with light-colored cats and those with no cats! It was suggested that darker colored cats have more antigens. But alas, another study found no difference. Some studies also indicate that long-haired cats shed fewer allergens than short-haired ones, but other studies found no difference. Such is the world of allergies.

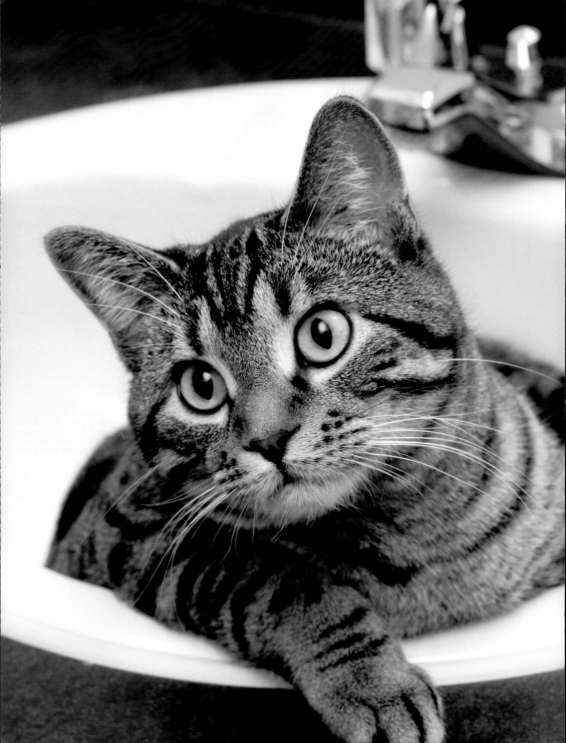

# KICK THE SNEEZE:
## Treatment and Management

**W**hile cat allergies are annoying, they are also controllable. In fact, they are probably easier to control than your cat, who, as you may have noticed, is not particularly interested in obeying you. Unless you are one of a handful of people on the planet who suffer an anaphylactic reaction when near one, you can keep your feline friend and manage your allergy. And by keeping the cat, I don't mean locking her out of the house to forage in the barn for wayward mice; I mean keeping her in the house with you.

way to control your allergy to cats is, surprisingly, to limit your exposure to *other* allergens. This is because allergies are cumulative; in other words, most folks who are allergic to one substance are usually allergic to others as well. And while it's hard to get away from allergens like dust and dust mites, others such as perfumes, soaps, paint, and mold can be more easily avoided.

In fact, many people allergic to cats are so slightly affected that the allergy itself is only provoked when they are exposed to other allergens at the same time. This is often referred to as an "allergy flare-up." In allergists' terms, this means that exposure to other allergens exceeds the sufferer's threshold level. So by minimizing your exposure to other allergens, you may be able to live more comfortably with your cat.

Many people allergic to cats are so slightly affected that the allergy itself is only provoked when they are exposed to other allergens as well.

## TREAT YOURSELF

The most efficient way to start treating your allergy is to treat yourself. After all, even if you completely rid your home of allergens, you have to go out into the world sometimes. The only constant in your life is you, so let's start there.

It is always wise to carefully evaluate any medication or treatment that you undertake. That goes for conventional, herbal, or any other type of treatment plan. The three big questions to ask are:

- Is it safe?
  - Is it effective?
    - Is it necessary?

Don't take any treatment unless you can answer "yes" to all three questions. Nowadays, many of us look online for medical information. But just because it's online doesn't mean that it is correct or safe. When researching, be sure that you know who is sponsoring the website. Universities, medical centers, government sources, and nonprofit research organizations are more credible than websites designed to sell you something. There is a difference between education and salesmanship. After you satisfy yourself that the information source is credible, make sure that the information is up to date. Nothing changes more quickly than medical news, and research is moving rapidly in this field.

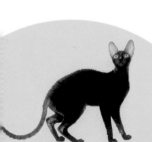

Allergies are very relative. Two people may be "allergic" to cats, but one of them can be as much as 100 times more allergic than the other. In addition, some people allergic to cats aren't even allergic to the Fel d1 protein, but rather to the albumin present in cat urine.

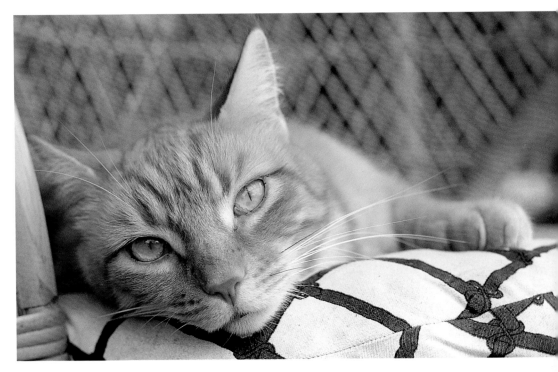

Beware of weasel words like "miracle cure" and "cures anything." There is no such cure. Good products are based on good science. Anecdotal evidence and testimonials are poor substitutes for real research.

*By minimizing your exposure to other allergens, like dust, mold, and pollen, you may be able to live more comfortably with your cat.*

## Allergen Immunotherapy

The most effective (and most expensive) way to treat an allergy is through allergen immunotherapy, which is a technical way of saying "allergy shots." Allergy shots have been available since 1911, although a lot of progress has been made in the last 100 years!

Additional information on asthma and other allergic diseases is available by calling the American College of Allergy, Asthma, and Immunology's (ACAAI) toll-free number (800) 842-7777 or visiting their website at www.acaai.org.

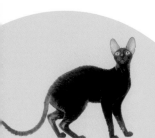

If you or your children are allergic to cats but can't bear the idea of living without one, explore getting desensitization shots before the arrival of the pet. Also known as immunotherapy injections, these shots can improve symptom severity, reduce the need for medication, and may even reduce your chances of developing new allergies in the future.

The purpose of allergen immunotherapy is to trick your system into producing blocking antibodies that will forestall an allergic response. After a while, the blood level of IgE antibodies (which cause most of the trouble) will also be reduced. This is a complex therapy, though, that must be undertaken under the supervision of your allergist.

In the first step in this process, the physician determines the villainous allergen through skin or serum testing. Once identified, he injects minuscule amounts of the subject material subcutaneously (beneath the skin). Your doctor will probably ask you to stay in the office for a period of time after receiving the injection simply to make sure that you do not have a reaction to it. A reaction can occur if too much of the allergen is injected too soon.

The amount of the allergen injected is gradually increased until you reach "maintenance level," which means that you no longer react to the allergen in the environment. At that point, you'll receive maintenance injections about once a week, at least at first. Later, their frequency can be reduced to once a month or once every six weeks. Some people are able to taper off of them entirely.

Allergen immunotherapy is not, as a rule, something that you want to hurry through. In rare cases, however, a bout of so-called "rush immunology" is deemed worth the risk. You might undergo this treatment if you must attend an event in which you simply can't avoid exposure to the allergen. Perhaps you're going to be given an award at a cat show, for example. This treatment regimen involves the injection of ever-increasing amounts of the allergen in a concentrated period, often only two or three days. If you do have a reaction, a quick antidote is available, so there's nothing to worry about. A mild reaction will respond to an antihistamine

## Immunotherapy

Treatment with immunotherapy usually takes from three to six months for complete effectiveness. Recent research reveals that once immunity is developed, patients continue to experience the benefits eight or more years after the shots have been discontinued. This is something that people who fear the expense might consider. Many allergy sufferers prefer to use over-the-counter drugs as a less expensive alternative. However, once you stop taking them, the symptoms do return. The biggest drawback to allergen immunotherapy is adverse reactions, which are rather common. However, serious reactions are very rare.

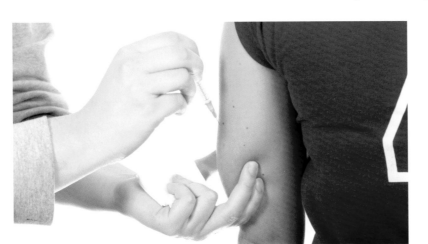

*The most efficient way to start treating your allergy is to treat yourself. You can visit an allergist or, if your symptoms aren't severe, try over-the-counter medications.*

like diphenhydramine to block the allergy symptoms. A more serious reaction may require epinephrine. All allergists' offices come fully stocked with both medications.

Immunotherapy is not for everyone. It can be expensive, and some people have such a dread of needles that they can't bring themselves to undergo it. It does not work for everyone, either, although research shows that people with pet allergies, especially cat allergies, respond extremely favorably to it; between 60 and 80 percent of people get complete relief from their symptoms. (People with dog allergies aren't quite so responsive, for some reason. Also, people with only occasional exposure tend to respond better than do pet owners.)

## THE ANTI-IgE ANTIBODY

New hope is always on the horizon. Researchers have developed the anti-IgE antibody (also called rhuMAb-E25 and omalizumab [Xolair]), available by prescription only. This is a monoclonal antibody to immunoglobulin E (IgE) developed to interfere early on in the allergy process by targeting the source of symptoms. It is a particularly useful therapy for asthmatic patients. By binding to circulating IgE in the blood, this antibody keeps IgE from binding to the mast cells and basophils, thus blocking the release of their inflammatory chemicals such as histamine and heparin. This early blockage is a departure from previous approaches that focus only on symptom relief and not on what causes them. However, omalizumab does not disassociate IgE already

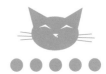

In one alternative treatment called enzyme potentiated desensitization, a very low dose of an allergen is mixed with a protein molecule (the enzyme beta-glucuronidase) and injected under the skin. It is somewhat like allergy shot treatment (immunotherapy), except a single injection is supposed to last a whole season. (As of yet, this therapy remains medically unproven.)

bound to effector cells. This is not a "rescue" medication and can't be used to treat sudden asthma attacks. It is a preventive only. The anti-IgE antibody is designed to be administered by injection every two to four weeks.

## An Allergy Vaccine?

Researchers at the Johns Hopkins University School of Medicine in Baltimore have recently conducted trials with an epitope vaccine developed from the cat dander allergen Fel d1. (An epitope, which is recognized by antibodies in the immune system, is the part of a protein responsible for a particular immune response.) The vaccine consisted of two 27-amino acid peptides derived from Fel d1 protein. A majority of the patients in the study (71 percent) who received four weekly injections showed improvements, and a follow-up study of the participants showed that 75 percent of those who had received the vaccine regimen continued to maintain some or all of their improvement after seven-and-a-half months.

If this therapy continues to prove successful, it will allow for the development of custom-designed anti-allergy treatments for many common allergens, perhaps all within a single under-the-skin injection.

## Medication

There are various forms of medication available to allergy sufferers, including many that do not require a prescription. The main types are:

*Allergen immunotherapy works by getting your body to produce "blocking antibodies" that prevent allergic responses like sneezing, wheezing, and sniffling.*

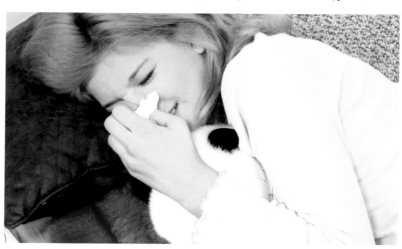

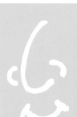

## Chimeras: Histamine Inhibitors

In April 2005, researchers at the University of California created a cat-human chimera (a mix of genetic material from both species). Specifically, they combined the Fel d1 protein (which, as we have seen, triggers allergic reactions) with a human protein that suppresses allergic reactions. The cat part of the protein binds to the immune cells that provoke the allergic reaction; the human part of the protein binds to the immune cells and instructs them to stop reacting. Because the human part dominates the cat part (unlike in real life), the allergic reaction is suppressed. The whole idea is to "retrain" the immune system. This injectable medication works by stopping the release of histamine, the natural chemical that causes allergy symptoms, including sneezing, wheezing, itching, and watery eyes.

One of the oddest things about the testing for this was that the tests were performed on mice who were allergic to cats. Mice have a lot of problems with cats, and allergies to them is not foremost. Researchers hope that similar products may work against a variety of allergens, including the deadly reactions that some people have to peanuts. We can only hope. So far the jury is out on this experiment.

- **Corticosteroids,** which help prevent and treat the inflammation associated with allergic conditions.
- **Antihistamines,** which block histamine, an inflammatory chemical released by the immune system during an allergic reaction.
- **Decongestants,** which relieve nasal and sinus congestion.
- **Leukotriene modifiers,** which block the effects of leukotrienes, more inflammatory chemicals released by your immune system during an allergic reaction.
- **Mast cell stabilizers,** which prevent the release of histamine.

Let's look at each of these in more detail.

## Corticosteroids

Other than some over-the-counter skin creams, corticosteroid medications are usually available by prescription only. They come in several forms: nasal sprays, eyedrops, skin creams, and pills or liquids.

Nasal sprays help prevent and relieve nasal stuffiness, sneezing, and an itchy, runny nose. Examples include budesonide (Rhinocort), mometasone (Nasonex), fluticasone (Flonase), and triamcinolone (Nasacort). While these medications aren't usually effective immediately, you may start to notice improvement after you've used them regularly for several days to two weeks. Nasal corticosteroids are generally safe for extended use.

Side effects may include an unpleasant smell or taste, and/or irritation, crusting, and bleeding in the nose, which may worsen in the winter when the air is drier. More serious (and rarer) side effects can include sinus

Because antihistamines are metabolized in the liver, people with liver disease should not take them.

damage and infection. As opposed to steroids taken by mouth or inhaled deeply through an inhaler or nebulizer, most nasal steroids don't seem to reduce bone density or affect growth in children. However, just to be safe, physicians usually prescribe the lowest effective dose.

Eyedrops are designed to relieve redness, tearing, and itching of the eyes. Examples include dexamethasone (Decadron, Dexair, and others), fluorometholone (Eflone, Fluor-Op, and others), and prednisolone (AK-Pred, Econopred, and others). Don't use eyedrops if you have glaucoma, an eye infection, or if you are pregnant. And if you wear contact lenses, you may want to switch to eyeglasses during treatment because corticosteroid eyedrops increase your risk of eye infection. Side effects may include blurred vision.

Skin creams are mostly used to relieve the scaling and itching caused by eczema (atopic dermatitis), an unusual but not unheard of result of cat allergies. Corticosteroid skin creams come in different strengths; low-potency creams include hydrocortisone (Allercort, Dermacort, and others); medium- to very high-potency skin creams include triamcinolone (Aristocort, Flutex, and others). The major side effects of skin creams are irritation and discoloration of the skin.

Pills and liquids (oral corticosteroids) like prednisone (Cordrol, Dexasone, and others) are sometimes used to treat severe allergy

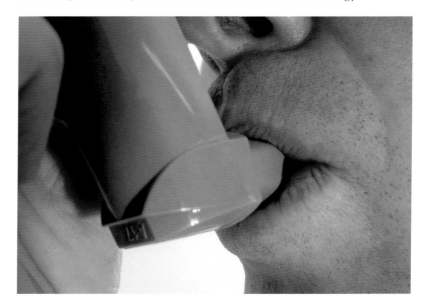

*Up to 40 percent of asthma sufferers show sensitivity to cats, so it's wise to limit their exposure.*

symptoms. Because the long-term use of these medications can cause severe side effects like cataracts, osteoporosis, and muscle weakness, they are usually only prescribed for short periods of time.

## Antihistamines

Histamines are the villains in many allergic responses. These inflammatory chemicals released by your immune system during an allergic reaction make your eyes red, your skin itch, your face swell, and your nose run (not a pretty combination).

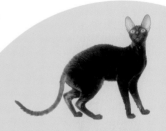

If histamines are the culprits, antihistamines are part of the answer. Antihistamines block the action of histamine. Blocking histamine reduces such symptoms as redness, swelling, runny nose, itchy, watery eyes, and hives (urticaria). This class of drugs was first developed in 1937. Many are available without a prescription, and they come in a variety of forms, including short acting and extended release.

Molecular biologists have cloned many major allergens and have identified the specific T-cell epitopes associated with the human immune response. These developments coincided with an increased understanding of allergic responses and the role that T-cells play in that response. Epitope vaccines were injected subcutaneously in very small doses. While the early indications were that a single injection could provide prolonged protection against a specific allergen, the long-term hope—if this project is ever resumed and further testing done—is that one or two injections will provide year-round protection.

Pills and liquids include diphenhydramine (Benadryl), chlorpheniramine (Chlor-Trimeton), and clemastine (Tavist). Because these older, first-generation antihistamines may make you drowsy, avoid using them before driving or doing anything else that requires intense concentration. Newer, second-generation antihistamines—such as loratadine (Claritin), which is available over the counter—are less likely to cause lethargy. Fexofenadine (Allegra) is a nonsedating prescription antihistamine. Another prescription antihistamine, cetirizine (Zyrtec), has an intermediate risk of causing sleepiness.

Nasal sprays include the prescription antihistamine azelastine (Astelin); it is effective for hay fever-like symptoms but may cause drowsiness.

Eyedrops available by prescription include emedastine (Emadine), levocabastine (Livostin), and olopatadine (Patanol). Side effects may include redness, tearing, headache, and stinging or burning. Like the corticosteroid eyedrops, antihistamine eyedrops increase the risk of eye inflammation for contact lens wearers, so it's better to wear glasses while taking treatment.

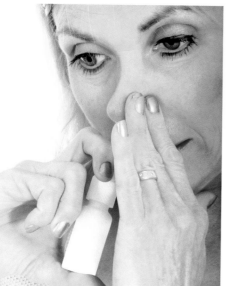

*Prescription nasal sprays are often helpful in controlling symptoms, and many have no side effects and are safe for children.*

## Did You Know?

To help stop tearing eyes, wet a washcloth with cold water and place it over your eyes for 15 to 20 minutes.

## Decongestants

Decongestants are formulated to relieve nasal and sinus congestion, as well as eye congestion caused by allergic conjunctivitis. Usually available over the counter, they come in various forms, including pills, liquids, sprays, and drops.

Pills and liquids usually contain pseudoephedrine (Sudafed, Actifed, and others), sometimes in combination with another drug. Medications such as Claritin-D, for example, combine pseudoephedrine with an antihistamine. Because oral decongestants raise blood pressure, avoid them if you have high blood pressure. Oral decongestants, especially those containing pseudophedrine, can also exacerbate the symptoms of prostate enlargement, making urination more difficult for some men.

Nasal sprays include phenylephrine (Neo-Synephrine) and oxymetazoline (Afrin). Don't use a decongestant nasal spray for more than a few days; after longer use, you may develop severe congestion as soon as you stop.

Eyedrops include tetrahydrozoline hydrochloride (Visine). While they are quite safe, your eyes may become persistently red if you overuse them.

## Leukotriene Modifiers

These drugs block the effects of leukotrienes, inflammatory chemicals released by your immune system during an allergic reaction. They have proven very effective in treating allergic asthma. Leukotriene modifiers are available by prescription only. They come in pill and chewable tablet form. Examples include montelukast (Singulair), zileuton (Zyflo), and zafirlukast (Accolate). The most common side effects include headache (montelukast) and nausea or upset stomach (zileuton) or a combination of both (zafirlukast).

## Mast Cell Stabilizers

Mast cell stabilizers actually prevent the release of histamine, not just stop it from binding to the cells in the mucous membranes the way antihistamines do. They may also reduce inflammation associated with hay fever and allergic conjunctivitis. Like other medications, they come in several forms.

Nasal sprays, including the over-the-counter medication cromolyn sodium (NasalCrom, Children's NasalCrom), have no serious side effects but may make the nasal passageways sting and burn, causing increased sneezing. Cromolyn sodium works best if you take it before your symptoms develop. Some people need to use the spray three or four times a day.

Eyedrops, available by prescription only, include cromolyn sodium (Crolom), lodoxamide (Alomide), pemirolast (Alamos), and nedocromil (Alocril). Cromolyn sodium and lodoxamide may make the eyes burn and sting, while pemirolast may cause chills, coughing, sneezing, and sore throat. Nedocromil may cause blurred vision or dry, itchy eyes. (Sometimes you just can't win.)

In most cases, the over-the-counter allergy medications work as well and are much cheaper than the prescription variety. The downside of these medications is that many cause drowsiness. However, a few of the newer prescription brands do not cause drowsiness because they do not penetrate the blood/brain barrier, and if sleepiness is a problem for you with most antihistamines, these might be worth inquiring about. Less frequent side effects (found mostly in older people) may include confusion, constipation, blurred vision, and in older men, problems urinating. If you have high blood pressure, over-the-counter antihistamines can be dangerous because they raise blood pressure and can lead to a heart attack or stroke, so seek advice from your doctor before using them.

Often, antihistamines are the first treatment for allergy symptoms, although sometimes a nasal decongestant is also used because they don't work well for congestion or tearing eyes. But be careful—don't use a nonprescription nasal decongestant for more than a few days. They are really designed just to help people with colds and are not for permanent

Reactions to airborne allergens tend to peak between 4 a.m. and 10 a.m., so it's advisable to take medications before bedtime.

## Medication Tips

- Keep all medication out of the reach of children and pets.
- Store medicines away from direct light and damp places.
- Don't keep outdated medicine or medicine that you no longer need. Dispose of it safely.
- Make sure to keep your allergy medications on hand, and refill prescriptions before the expiration dates.
- Use medications as prescribed, but don't wait for symptoms to get out of hand.

allergy sufferers. After a few days of using them, you may get a rebound effect, and your nose may become even more congested than before.

## Complementary and Alternative Treatments

You are not restricted to conventional medicine to cure your allergies. Other modalities such as acupuncture, homeopathy, herbal remedies, and hypnosis, for example, have been used for hundreds of years to control symptoms or even get at the source of allergies. These methods have had varying success rates, as has conventional Western medicine. For most people, the best choices are an allergist and the local drug store, but many people have had better luck using alternative medicine. Some "conventional" doctors also advocate the use of alternative therapies, which doesn't lessen the confusion any, believe me.

### Chinese Medicine: Acupuncture, Acupressure, and Herbs

*You are not restricted to conventional medicine to cure your allergies. Alternative treatments are also available such as acupuncture, acupressure, and herbal remedies.*

Traditional Chinese medicine has its origin in ancient Taoist philosophy, which views a person as an energy system in which the body and mind are unified, each influencing and balancing the other. The energy is called Qi (pronounced *chee*). Qi is a broad term for all the body's energies: electrical, chemical, magnetic, and radiant. This energy is said to circulate throughout the body along specific pathways that are called meridians. Each one of these rivers of energy flows through and influences an internal organ. If the flow of energy is blocked, the system is disrupted and a disease occurs.

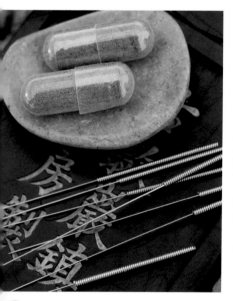

The most powerful points on these meridians lie on the arms and legs below the elbows and knees. The most powerful ones, which are on the extremity of each channel, are called the five Shu points. They are compared to the flow of water and named the source points, well points, stream points, river points, and sea points.

Also, according to Chinese medical theory, disease is an imbalance of some sort within the body. The imbalance can be any of these:

**Excess/Deficiency:** Too much or too little of something. Sudden onset problems are considered to be

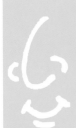

## Chinese Herbal Remedy

A study in the September 2004 issue of the journal *Allergy* concluded that a combination of Chinese herbs and weekly acupuncture sessions may be effective at relieving the symptoms of seasonal allergic rhinitis. Along with acupuncture, patients using traditional Chinese medicine (TCM) received a basic herbal formula (consisting of schizonepeta, chrysanthemum, cassia seed, plantago seed, and tribulus). They were instructed to take it as a decoction (mash) three times per day parallel to acupuncture treatment. In addition to the basic formula, every patient received a second formula tailored to the patient's individual TCM diagnosis. The acupuncture–herb combination appeared to be well tolerated by patients in both groups. Two patients complained of pain due to needle insertion. Five patients (two TCM, three control) complained that the herbal decoction either tasted bitter or made them feel nauseous. However, none of the patients experienced "severe or serious adverse events" that caused them to leave the trial.

caused by excess; chronic problems by deficiency. Symptoms of excess are usually stronger than those of deficiency.

**Inside/Outside:** This refers to whether the originating problems come from outside the body (as with allergies) or from inside. Of course, allergens can invade the body and become interior over time.

**Hot/Cold:** This refers to the way in which the disease affects the body, basically as fevers or chills.

**Damp/Dry:** Swollen tissues, phlegm, and fluids are caused by dampness. Fevers and scratchy throats are instances of dryness.

## Acupuncture

This technique is said to bring fast relief from nasal congestion, discharge, and itching. Using very fine needles, acupuncture stimulates the nervous system to release chemicals that influence the body's internal regulating system. The improved energy and biochemical balance produced by acupuncture results in the stimulation of the body's natural healing abilities. Acupuncture can help to strengthen the body's resistance and can regulate antigen–antibody reactions. This is important in helping to relieve hay fever and other allergic responses such as asthma.

During a therapy session, the practitioner places very thin, sterile, stainless steel acupuncture needles into points on congested areas of the face, as well as into corresponding acupuncture points on the arms and legs. The stimulation of the points helps to decongest the sinuses and mucous membranes. These points also may be treated with warming by the Chinese herb, moxa, or by stimulating the needles with a mild, painless electric charge at the tip. While results vary from patient to patient, many

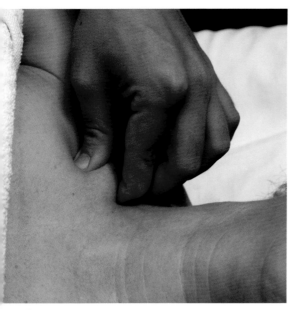

*Acupressure is given on pressure points to stimulate the flow of energy and improve circulation throughout the body to treat disease or improve health.*

report feeling immediate relief from congestion and coughs. And some studies show that people have lower levels of the allergy-related antibody IgE in their blood after therapy.

## Acupressure

An ancient Chinese total body treatment, acupressure is given on pressure points to stimulate the flow of energy and improve circulation throughout the body. This treatment is based on the premise that channels (or meridians) of energy (Qi) flowing throughout the body may be manipulated by pressure to treat disease or improve health. It is hypothesized that blockage of the energy channels results in disease, including allergy. Unlike acupuncture, acupressure requires no needles, relying instead on the thumbs, palms, heels of the hands, and elbows to apply pressure to vital points on the body to release blockages. The patient can remain dressed during this procedure.

## Chinese Herbs

Since time immemorial, people have used herbs and dietary changes or additions to fight allergies. Most of these have had no scientific studies to back them up. One common herbal concoction used included ephedra, which was eventually banned by the FDA in 2003. However, that doesn't mean that all herbal remedies are dangerous—and after all, plenty of "approved" FDA drugs have been removed from the market as well. Every Chinese herb has its own attributes, which include its energy, its flavor, its movement, and its related meridians or channels. Herbs are quite a study in and of themselves, but here are the basics related to allergy.

From a Chinese point of view, allergic rhinitis is caused by a deficiency of the lung and kidney's defensive-Qi systems, combined with retention of chronic "wind" in the nose. You may note that the terminology seems strange. Some modern practitioners take these colorful terms metaphorically.

According to traditional Chinese medicine, the liver (always) and lung systems (sometimes) are malfunctioning in allergy cases. Liver system imbalances produce watery eyes, headache, itchy throat, and itchy nose. Lung system imbalances produce coughing, wheezing, sneezing, and nonitchy skin disorders.

One classic Chinese herbal remedy for allergy treatment contains the following herbs (with the common English name, Latin or scientific name, and Chinese name, in that order, along with the amount prescribed and the herb's effects):

- **Angelica Root** (*Angelica Dahurica*, Bai Zhi, 75 mg)
  Expels wind, releases surface, alleviates pain, reduces swelling, expels dampness, and alleviates discharge.
- **Magnolia Bud** (*Magnolia Flos*, Xin Ye Hua, 75 mg)
  Expels wind, relieves surface, opens nasal passages.
- **Anemarrhena Root** (*Anemarrhena Radix*, Zhi Mu, 75 mg)
  Clears heat, quells fire, nurtures Yin, moistens the dry.
- **Centipede Plant** (*Centepeda Herba*, Shi Hu Sui, 75 mg)
  Dissolves phlegm, expels wind, disperses cold, removes damp, removes film.
- **Patchouli Plant** (*Agastach Pogostemi*, Huo Xiang, 75 mg)
  Transforms dampness, releases the exterior, harmonizes the center, expels dampness.
- **Liquidambar Fruit** (*Liquidambar Fructus*, Lu Lu Tong, 75 mg)
  Promotes the flow of Qi and blood, unblocks the channels, opens the "middle burner."
- **Cocklebur Fruit** (*Xanthium Fructus*, Cang Er Zi, 75 mg)
  Opens the nasal passages, disperses wind, expels dampness, relieves itching.
- **Sicklepod Seed** (*Cassia Torre Sm.* Ju Ming Zi, 37.5 mg)
  Clears the vision, expels wind heat, benefits the eyes, clears the liver.
- **Mint Leaf** (*Herba Mentha*, Bo He, 37.5 mg)
  Clears the head and eyes, benefits the throat, disperses wind heat, encourages the flow of liver Qi.
- **Siler Root** (*Ledebouriella Rx*, Fang Feng, 37.5 mg)
  Releases the exterior, expels wind, alleviates pain.
- **Hairy Sage** (*Hb. Schizonepeta*, Jing Jie, 37.5 mg)
  Releases the exterior, expels wind heat and wind cold, alleviates itching.

Always wash your hands after petting the cat or after handling her bedding and toys. And as much as possible, keep your hands away from your eyes, nose, and mouth afterward because they are the pathways to the inner you.

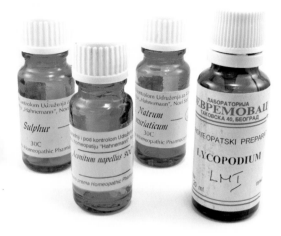

*Homeopathic remedies made from natural substances are believed to work by stimulating the body's own healing processes.*

- **Mulberry Root Bark** (*Cortex Mori Albae Radices*, Sang Bai Pi, 37.5 mg) Clears heat from the lungs, reduces edema.
- **Tree Peony Root Bark** (*Cortex Moutan Radicis*, Mu Dan Pi, 37.5 mg) Clears heat, cools blood, invigorates blood, reduces swelling, clears ascending liver fire.

## Chiropractic Care

Although chiropractic is not a treatment for allergies per se, its proponents claim that by permitting the nervous system to function with less stress, the immune system will function more effectively. Chiropractic therapy frees up the nerves so that they are not irritated and hypersensitive to stimuli.

## Homeopathy

Developed by Samuel Hahnemann in the 18th century, homeopathy is a system of medicine that is based on the Law of Similars: like cures like. (The word "homeopathy" comes from two Greek words that mean "like disease.") A holistic approach to treatment, this system is based on the idea that substances that produce symptoms of illness in healthy people will have a curative effect when given in very dilute quantities to sick people who have the same symptoms. The remedies made from these substances are believed to work by stimulating the body's own healing processes.

Homeopathic medications or remedies are made by homeopathic pharmacies in accordance with the processes described in the Homeopathic Pharmacopoeia of the United States (HPUS). The substances used may be made from plants, animals, or even minerals and are considered nontoxic. They are diluted carefully until very little of the original remains, and then they are strongly shaken, a process known as succussion. The number following the medication indicates the number of times that the substance has been diluted. The more diluted the substance is, the stronger the medicine. (This goes against common sense, but in homeopathy, succussion releases the healing energy from the substance.)

Although the efficacy of homeopathic medicine has not been proven, a study conducted by doctors at Glasgow University showed that patients with allergic hay fever-like symptoms were tested with positive results. Half were given a homeopathic remedy based on extracts from various allergy-causing substances. The other half were simply given a placebo, although, because of the dilution, the chemical formula of the two liquids appeared to be identical. The patients given the homeopathic remedy experienced a significant improvement in their nasal symptoms—their noses were far clearer. On average, the homeopathy patients were 22 percent better, while the placebo group was only 2.5 percent better. The results with the homeopathic treatment are roughly similar to those that a doctor might expect to achieve with a steroid nasal spray. However, homeopathy appears to have no side effects at all.

The following homeopathic remedies are recommended for pet allergies:

- **Adrenalinum** (Adrenaline) 6X
- **Allium Cepa** (Red Onion) 6X
- **Arsenicum Iodatum** (Arsenious Iodide) 6X
- **Euphrasia Officinalis** (Eyebright) 6X
- **Sabadilla** (Cevadilla) 6X
- **Silicea** (Silica) 6X
- **Hair and dander extracts:** Cat 12X (Hair only).

## NAET (Nambudripad's Allergy Elimination Techniques)

NAET combines kinesiology (muscle responsive testing), chiropractic, and oriental medicine to clear allergic reactions through a reprogramming of the brain, according to its proponents. Its effectiveness has not been proven.

## Herbal and Dietary Supplements

The new rage in herbal allergy therapies is the European herb butterbur (*Petasites hybridus*). In one study, published in the *British Medical Journal*, a group of Swiss researchers showed how just one tablet of butterbur four times daily was as effective as a popular antihistamine drug in controlling symptoms of hay fever without the traditional side effect of drowsiness that sometimes occurs.

Did You Know?

Homeopathy appears to have no side effects.

Other herbal supplements proving helpful may include freeze-dried nettles and a tonic made from the herb goldenseal, which may be added to a saline (salt water) nasal spray.

Some additives that have been touted as curing or treating allergies include:

- **Bitter Orange (*citrus aurantium*).** A natural extract, bitter orange is on the FDA's Generally Recognized As Safe (GRAS) list. However, this substance is similar to ephedra in some respects and therefore may pose similar health risks when used in supplements or herbal remedies.
- **Calcium and Magnesium.** Calcium and magnesium are important nutrients for the allergy sufferer. They help to relax an overreactive nervous system. These minerals help to manage the stresses on the body caused by allergic reactions.
- **Co-enzyme Q10.** This natural substance stimulates immune system function and works as a powerful antioxidant. It moves energy throughout the body, increasing the efficiency of cellular metabolism, and it is also beneficial in combating allergies, asthma, and lowered immunity. Co-enzyme Q10 is found in all healthy tissues in the body.
- **Echinacea.** This herb stimulates the immune system and may also protect against infection and stimulate tissue repair and healing.
- **Fatty Acids.** Essential fatty acids like omega 3 and 6 (ones that we can't produce ourselves) are important to the immune system because they reduce inflammation associated with allergic responses by aiding in the production of prostaglandins, hormone-like substances that counter inflammation.
- **Grape Seed Extract.** Grape seed extract is derived from the seeds or skins of grapes and is believed to have natural antihistamine and anti-inflammatory properties.
- **Pycnogenol.** An extract of maritime pine trees, this substance is believed to have anti-inflammatory properties.
- **Quercetin.** This flavenoid compound is found in some fruit and plants. It is believed to have properties that enhance the skin's elasticity and can inhibit allergic reactions. It may even control the release of histamine. The good news is that quercetin is plentiful in red wine.
- **Spirulina.** A class of algae that grows in warm climates all over the world, spirulina may also have antihistamine properties.

**Did You Know?**

Herbal products can interact with each other or with other medications. Check with your doctor before using them.

- **Sulfur.** Sulfur aids in the treatment of allergies, both environmental (house dust, animal hair, etc.) and those associated with food and drugs. People who are allergic to certain foods or who have reactions to medications (nonsteroidal anti-arthritic medications and antibiotics) show either a decreased reaction or a complete tolerance to the particular foods or medications when taking sulfur.

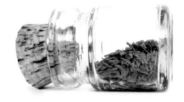

- **Thymus Extract.** The thymus is part of the immune system. It comprises two lobes lying just below the thyroid gland and above the heart. The thymus is responsible for many immune system functions, including the production of T lymphocytes, a type of white blood cell responsible for cell-mediated immunity, which are mechanisms not controlled or mediated by antibodies. Cell-mediated immunity is also critical in protecting against allergies. Thymus extracts used as nutritional supplements are most often derived from young calves. This extract has been shown effective in preventing recurrent upper respiratory tract infections and in relieving allergies.

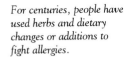

*For centuries, people have used herbs and dietary changes or additions to fight allergies.*

- **Vitamin C.** Vitamin C's natural antihistamine properties make it a classic allergy treatment. A daily dose of 1,000 to 4,000 milligrams may help to reduce the severity of sinus stuffiness and runny nose.

None of these herbal remedies has been proven to work as well as conventional methods, but some people swear by them. One old folk medication suggests swallowing a spider. That may work, too. Then again, maybe it won't.

## Buying Herbs

Because there are few federal regulations regarding herbs, it's mostly buyer beware, although a few private sector groups have made some attempts to regulate and rate them. These organizations include the US Pharmacopoeia, ConsumerLab.com, *Good Housekeeping,* and NSF International. Of these, only the *Good Housekeeping* program requires a product to prove that it's both safe and effective. To obtain this certification, a manufacturer must submit research-based evidence that the product does what it claims to do and that it does so without harming the consumer. Look for this type of information on product labels.

Speaking of labels, every label on an herbal supplement should include the following information:

- Its common and Latin (scientific) name—for example, feverfew (*Tanacetum parthenium*). It may also include the part of the herb used (leaf, root, seed).
- Net quantity of contents—for example, 60 capsules.
- Ingredients and amounts.
- Disclaimer: "This substance has not been evaluated by the Food and Drug Administration. This product is not intended to diagnose, treat, cure, or prevent any disease."
- Supplement facts panel, which includes serving size, amount, and active ingredient.
- Other ingredients, such as herbs and amino acids, for which no daily values have been established.
- Name and address of the manufacturer, packer, or distributor.

As with any medication, herbal products can interact with each other or with other conventional medications (both prescription and over the counter). People with liver problems, high blood pressure, diabetes, or elderly patients, children, and pregnant or nursing women should be extra careful.

Avoid any wild gathered herb. It could have been sprayed with powerful road pesticides or urinated on, or it might be endangered from overgathering, as happened with goldenseal.

## Hypnosis

Hypnosis is an induced form of deep relaxation in which a patient is susceptible to suggestions from the practitioner. It may work to help people stick to their anti-allergy regimen (like vacuum regularly, keep the cat out of the bedroom, etc.) and may also work to help relieve stress and thus strengthen the immune system.

## CHILDREN AND ALLERGIES

The connection between pets and childhood allergies is unclear, with various studies showing different results. Some suggest that very early exposure to animals may reduce the chances that a child will develop allergies later in life.

One such study conducted in 2006 by Dr. Esmeralda Morales of the University of Arizona, Tucson, examined 486 children from birth to one year of age. While children growing up in dog-owning households appeared to have some slight protection from itchy allergies, children in cat-owning homes appeared to be more at risk for the condition.

But something odd also turned up in the study. Previous studies, including one done in Sweden in 2001, showed that having cats and dogs in the household seemed to offer protection against allergic diseases. In that study, 412 youngsters were tested for allergies at 7 years of age and again at age 12. Of those children living in petless homes during their first year, nearly 9 percent developed asthma, compared to only 3 percent who were exposed to pets. Allergies also developed in nearly 9 percent of children in the no-pet group, while only 6 percent of the pet-exposed children did.

A larger study also done in Sweden in 2003 by allergist Thomas Platts-Mills of the University of Virginia, along with fellow Swedish researchers, tested 2,500 children and found that the longer children had pets—ideally, beginning during their first two years—the lower their frequency of having pet allergies. Children who continually owned pets were less likely to have pet dander allergies than new pet owners or those who had been briefly exposed only earlier in life. In fact, of those who were proven to be allergic to cats, 80 percent had never had a cat at home. A study in 2002 found that babies raised in a home with two or more dogs or cats were up to 77

*People with allergic parents are much more likely to develop allergies themselves, although the connection between pets and childhood allergies is unclear.*

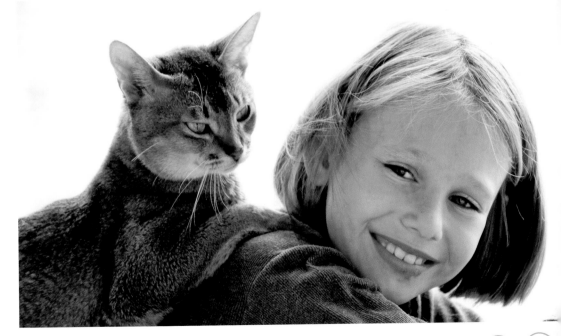

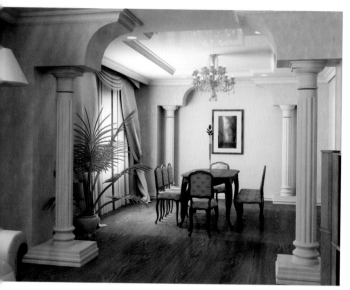

*When you suffer from allergies, remove any materials in your home that will collect allergens like dust and mold; for example, hardwood floors are better than carpeting.*

percent less likely to develop various types of allergies at age 6 than kids raised without pets. The protective effect worked not only against pet dander allergies but against other kinds as well, such as dust mites, ragweed, and grass. One explanation is that early high pet allergen exposure may lead to changes in the immune system so that it is less likely to produce an allergic response.

Dennis R. Ownby, chief of Allergy and Immunology at the Medical College of Georgia, studied 474 children from birth to age 7. He discovered that children exposed to two or more indoor pets were less than half as likely to develop allergies—not just to pet secretions but also to ragweed, dust mites, and grass. Ownby theorizes that the licks children receive when playing with their pets transfer enough gram-negative bacteria to change the way the child's immune system responds. However, be forewarned: Parents who smoke wipe out the anti-allergy benefits that their infants receive from early pet exposure.

The jury is still out, and in many cases none of the findings seem strong enough to determine for sure whether having a cat is ultimately harmful or beneficial. When you consider the emotional pluses of owing a cat, the answer seems clear—at least to the cat lovers of the world.

## TREAT THE HOUSE

### Reduce Dander-Catchers

When you suffer from allergies, it's important to remove any materials in your home that will trap or collect dander and any other allergy-provoking substances such as dust and mold.

### Carpets

One of the most effective methods of keeping a house free of allergen-loaded cat dander is to remove carpeting. Everything that flies in the air lands sooner or later, and gravity dictates that a great deal of it will land on your carpet. And once it's there, it tends to stay there, no matter how much you vacuum. Cat allergen particles are so minuscule that they can filter through the rug and deposit themselves in the pad beneath it. It seems to be a law of nature (almost) that the more carpet you have, the more dander you'll collect.

Much better choices would be hardwood flooring, ceramic or vinyl tiles, or linoleum. Although they also collect dander, they don't soak up urine and smell. There is no reliable way to remove the urine smell permanently from a carpet or the pad beneath it, but it's easy to wash the other flooring options to remove allergens.

If you absolutely must have carpeting, buy a brand that is coated with Teflon. Otherwise, if possible, choose one with natural rather than artificial fibers. Artificial fibers seem to capture and hold on to allergic particles much more.

If you do have wall-to-wall carpeting—possibly the worst type of carpeting for pet owners—you will need to steam clean it frequently, at least every two months. For best results in removing allergens, try using a good commercial product such as Allersearch X-Mite Carpet Solution. This rug shampoo deactivates allergens created by dust mites, household pets, cat dander, and even certain pollens while simultaneously cleaning and refreshing velvet, velour, corduroy, carpets, and all other pile fabrics.

## Window Treatments and Furniture

Like carpets, other things like curtains, blinds, and furniture also collect allergens. If possible, replace fabric-upholstered furniture with nonporous material like wood or leather.

You should also get rid of curtains and replace them with contemporary vertical blinds, which are easier to keep clean. If you are addicted to fabric window treatments, choose the sort that are easily taken down, thrown in the laundry, and replaced. Do this every month. (Demite is an excellent anti-allergy detergent.)

Don't forget to damp-dust frequently, including places that you might normally forget—the tops of refrigerators, high shelves, and the like. You can bet there is dander floating around up there. It also helps to use a duster that creates a static charge, such as Swiffers or Pledge Grab-It products, which allow more dust to be removed. For dusting furniture, you can purchase a magnetic wiping fabric that can be used on

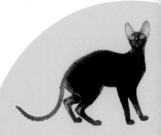

One way to make your cleaning chores a bit more manageable is to stock and organize a closet full of all your grooming and cleaning supplies. This is a lot easier than having everything scattered all over the house.

wood, metal, glass, plastic, ceramic, and television or computer screens. Simply wipe lightly. Wash the magnetic fabric with a mild detergent.

While you are doing all that, wash down the walls, too. Even walls can collect allergens. Between washings, take a long-handled brush and wipe them down every other week.

## Bedroom Items

Allergy sufferers should not use feather pillows or down comforters. If you can't live without a feather pillow, encase it in a plastic or cloth casing with a zipper so that none of the feathers can escape. A microfiber fill is an excellent choice.

Cover your mattress with a vinyl cover and change all bedding (including blankets and quilts) at least once a week. Be aware that vinyl can break down after several years of use, so membrane-free allergy relief bedding may be a better choice. The average bed has between 1 and 10 million dust mites. It's not a pretty picture.

You can even buy a mattress cover with pore sizes of 6 microns. While this does let animal dander through, it will stop dust mites, and 80 percent of cat allergy sufferers are also allergic to dust mites. By removing this

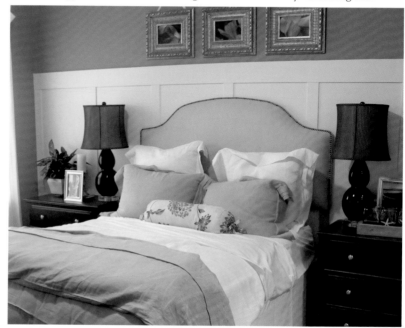

*Do not use feather pillows or down comforters, and keep the bedroom free of clutter.*

allergen from your environment, you will sleep easier and build up your resistance to cat dander. Remember, allergies are cumulative!

Keep the bedroom free of piles of books, too, because they collect dust like mad and are probably full of cat dander.

## Install Air Filters and Cleaners

While fresh air is a wonderful commodity, the stuff that issues forth from your furnace vent may leave much to be desired. These air currents simply distribute allergens throughout the entire house. It does little good to contain a cat in one room if her dander is floating around everywhere during heating and air-conditioning seasons. Yet another reason to save energy! Put on a sweater or stick your feet in a bucket of cold water. You'll be surprised to find how relaxing that is. I'm kidding (sort of), of course. However, there are steps you can take to lessen the dander-carrying capacity of your central air and heating systems.

Invest in a high-efficiency particular air (HEPA) filter for the central air/heating system, which will remove airborne allergens. You can also put an electronic air cleaner in every room in your house that includes a HEPA filter. Use these for at least four hours every day. This simple step can remove a large percentage of pet allergens from the circulating air in your home. However, these devices are designed to remove only airborne particles, not those that have already enmeshed themselves into furniture and carpets. To get the best results from your HEPA, be sure that you have taken all the steps necessary to get rid of the dander already accumulated first.

Choosing the proper HEPA to purchase depends on a multitude of factors, including the size of the space in which the unit will be placed, the number of times per hour the air will be completely cycled, and the size of the particles that the system can handle (the smaller the better). Remember that animal dander is a mere 2.5 microns (1 micron = 1/25,000 inch). Maintenance of the units is equally important. Change the filters frequently. Some good choices for allergy-free electrostatic filters are the 3M Disposable Electrostatic Central Furnace Filter, the Taskmaster Healthmate, and the Pleat-a-Static.

You can also use a room air purifier as an extra measure in the bedroom to remove airborne animal dander. Make sure that the exhaust from the air cleaner is not directed toward rugs or upholstered furnishings so as not to shake loose allergens that may have settled there.

**Did You Know?**

Because pets stir up dust, having dogs and cats may also aggravate dust mite allergies in people at risk to them.

*To remove airborne allergens like dander, install high-efficiency air filters in air/heating systems, maintain air ducts and replace filters, and vacuum regularly.*

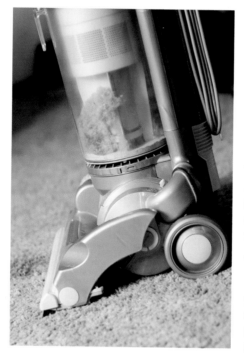

Maintaining and filtering air ducts is also important. Choose high-quality pleated electrostatic filters, and change them monthly or as directed. These prevent the spread of dust, mold spores, and dander throughout the duct system's point of entry. The Vent-ProHeating Filter is a good choice. Many people find the permanent, washable electrostatic models even more effective.

### Vacuum Often

Your vacuum cleaner is your best friend if you have allergies, but your old standby may not be good enough. Use a model that has a HEPA filter or double filter. Look for a tight-sealed vacuum system with at least an S-class filter that meets the US HEPA standard of removing 99.97 percent of all particles 0.3 microns or larger. Cat dander gets smaller than this, but you need to work with the best technology available. You can rest assured that a HEPA filter will effectively trap all the household allergens picked up by your vacuum cleaner. Allergic people benefit most from using models with bags; if you have a bagless vacuum, get someone else to change the bag for you. Change the vacuum bags frequently—do not wait until they are full. Follow up vacuuming with a spray such as Allersearch ADS Anti-Allergen Dust Spray to denature the remaining allergens.

Avoid perfumed air fresheners and cleaners because they can cause allergic reactions.

### Use Air Conditioners and Fans

When operating an air conditioner, choose the "circulate" setting for both home and car air-conditioning systems. This will prevent animal dander allergens from entering from outside. Avoid ceiling fans because they simply stir up the dander.

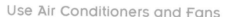

Also, clean window air-conditioning units and humidifiers often to eliminate mold and mildew growth.

## Lower the Humidity

Reduce the humidity in your home below 45 percent. This simple step reduces mold growth, to which you also may be allergic. To measure the humidity level, you can buy an inexpensive hygrometer, which is available at your local hardware or discount store.

## Dry the Bathroom

Install dehumidifiers in bathrooms, basements, and other places in the house where molds tend to collect. Dry out the basin and tub after use. They collect mold (even if you can't see it). Wash shower curtains and bathroom tiles with mold-killing products. Reducing all allergens will help you deal with your cat allergy.

*Run the furnace or central air-conditioning fan continuously for at least two hours after vacuuming to remove allergens that may have been stirred up into the air from the carpeting.*

## Open the Windows (Maybe)

Just opening the windows on a breezy day will help clear your home of dander. You can also use a fan to push stale, dander-laden air out the window. However, if you are allergic to pollens (April through May), grasses (June through July), or ragweed (August through October), keeping the window shut may be your only option. (There is no ragweed out West, so Californians are safe.) There are also tree allergies, the most common from maple, ash, oak, elm, birch, and cedar.

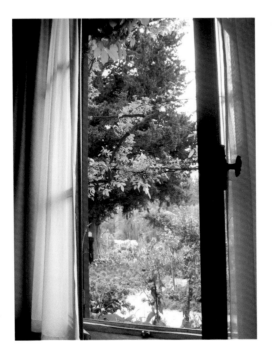

*Opening the windows can help clear your home of dander; however, if you're allergic to pollen, grasses, or trees, avoid doing so during allergy season.*

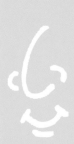

## Cat Litter

Most people who are allergic to cats are also allergic to other things, one of the most common being dust. That being so, it behooves the wise (and allergic) cat owner to take special care in choosing a litter that will reduce his or her chances of an allergic reaction. (It doesn't do the cat any good either.)

If possible, select an unscented litter rather than one "enriched" by perfumes or deodorizers that really do nothing more than mask the smell. If you must clean the litter box yourself, wear a dust mask while doing so (and do it daily), and pour the litter slowly to keep dust from spreading.

The fine dust from conventional, coarse-grained clay cat litter can aggravate allergies. Always choose a clumping litter, most of which are free of dust. Another excellent idea is a product is modestly called "The World's Best Cat Litter." This litter is made not from clay or artificial materials, but from whole kernel corn. It clumps, is easily scooped, and it's flushable. (It is safe for septic tanks as well and can be use in "self-cleaning" litter boxes.) It lasts longer than traditional clay litters, too. It is 99 percent dust free.

### Avoid Aerosols and Sprays

Avoid using aerosols, sprays, paints, insecticides, chemicals, epoxy, and heavy air fresheners in the house. And of course, ban smoking in the home. These irritants trigger allergy symptoms and compound the effects of allergens such as pet dander, dust mites, and pollen.

### Experiment with Antidander Products

Several companies produce excellent antidander products such as Allerpet, a spray that you can use on your home and even on the dog or cat! Various types of disposable wipes developed by pet product companies provide a quick and easy way to remove loose fur from furniture (or even from the cat). Those rolling lint picker-uppers work well also.

### Restrict Access

Your cat doesn't need to have unlimited access to every available living or sleeping space in your home. Cats rule, but there needs to be a system of checks and balances! Keep her off furniture (especially upholstered furniture) and out of certain rooms—especially your bedroom, whether you are in it or not. Research shows that if you can breathe eight to ten hours of "pure" air every night, you can tolerate more exposure to allergic substances during the day. The bedroom, especially, should be free of clutter. Remove magazines, books and newspapers, rugs, drapes, junk under the bed, and so on. The more washable surfaces there are, the better.

In rare cases, repeated flare-ups of allergy attacks in children can cause lung damage. In situations like this, you may be forced to find your cat another home if you can't bring your child's symptoms under control.

If you do allow the cat on the couch (and it's not that easy to keep her off), at least cover it with a sheet and wash the sheet every day. The sheet will collect much of the dander.

Use a towelette or moist wipe to remove dirt, mud, and other grime or potential allergens from your pet's paws before she can track them inside the house.

### Provide an Outside Room

Many people build outdoor enclosed areas for their cats. The animals enjoy the fresh air and bird watching, and you get some additional time in a catless house. But remember that catless is not danderless— unfortunately, some allergens hang around even when the cat is outside. Cats can make their presence known, although they themselves are not actually there. It's part of their magic.

### Wash Toys and Bedding

Wash all your cat's toys and bedding frequently in very hot, soapy water. Bedding should be covered in allergen-resistant plastic. You can

*Your pets don't need to have unlimited access to the entire house. Keep cats out of the bedroom (where we spend a third of our time) and, more importantly, off the bed.*

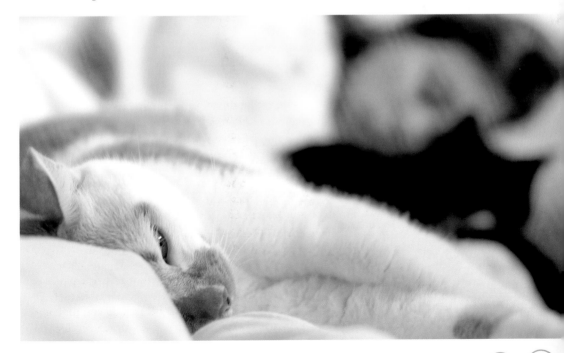

even buy an allergen-resistant pet bed made from "breathable" Cordura nylon, a washable fabric tougher than cotton or fleece that traps dust and other allergy-causing particles.

### Protect Your Car

If you travel with your cat (and that includes going to the vet), you can be sure that there is cat dander in your car, even if the cat is properly kept in her traveling crate. It helps to put a washable covering over the seat that will collect the dander. Launder the cover when you return home.

## TREAT THE CAT—DON'T GET HER DANDER UP!

One of the best ways to keep yourself from suffering allergic symptoms is to take excellent care of your cat. Anything that injures or irritates her skin can result in the production of more dander. As an allergy sufferer, you will know that something may be wrong with your cat if you start sneezing more!

Careful grooming is the first step. This doesn't mean that you have to do it yourself—by all means get your spouse, friend, child, or groomer to do it for you. Allergies can be good for something!

### Bathing

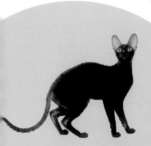

I know that it is difficult, but please do not hug or kiss your cat if you suffer from cat dander allergies. Most cats aren't that crazy about being kissed anyway. They won't miss it a bit.

Frequent, thorough bathing is an excellent way to remove dead hair and dander from your cat. Research has shown that washing a pet two to three times a week can remove up to 84 percent of the surface allergens and significantly reduce the amount of future allergens produced. Dirty cats can develop raw, irritated skin that simply makes them want to lick more and thus distribute allergen-containing saliva all over their fur.

When bathing your cat, use cool, distilled water. This may reduce allergen levels. If you use a quality shampoo with a good conditioner (as you do with your own hair), you can bathe your cat several times a week. It won't hurt her in the least; in fact, her skin and coat will glow!

There are several good pet products on the market. One is a clear, nontoxic, deodorizing plant-based shampoo that denatures protein allergens on contact. It also helps to control fleas and ticks. Be sure that the shampoo you use is a moisturizing one. Dry skin is itchy and flaky, and that's a bad combination for allergy sufferers. There are special

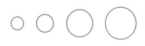
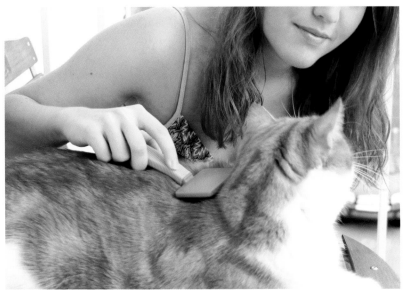

*One of the best ways to keep yourself from suffering allergic symptoms is to take excellent care of your cat. Regular grooming is the first step.*

products available such as Allergy Relief Center pet shampoo. You can even make a homemade shampoo that works perfectly well: Combine small amounts of a gentle, liquid dishwashing soap, white vinegar, and glycerin. Baby shampoo works well, too.

While it's not fun to bathe a cat, it's not the horror show that most people think it is. Grasp your cat firmly by the nape of the neck while washing; keep a firm grip. Again, it's best if you can get someone else to do this for you. If you are also allergic to grass or pollen and happen to have an outside cat, you might need to bathe her after she's been outside running around.

## Brushing

Brushing is another way to remove dead hair and stimulate the skin so that it remains in great condition, neither dry nor greasy. Frequent brushing helps to distribute oils through the coat and to reduce dander.

Always wear a mask and protective gloves when grooming your pet. Don't hesitate to beg or hire someone else to do it—sticking your nose in cat hair isn't likely to help your allergy. Use gentle strokes, and avoid using any grooming tools that irritate the skin.

After grooming or playing with your cat, remove your clothing, which is now full of animal dander, and wash it. Keep these clothes out of the

Spray your cat between baths with a moisturizer (humectant) to keep the dander down.

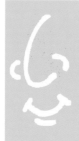

## Cat Bath

A new study done at the University of Virginia Asthma and Allergic Diseases Center in Charlottesville, Virginia has indicated that frequently bathing your cat could reduce the shedding of allergy-irritating proteins (Fel d1). Cats washed with soap, water, and a hose had a 44 percent decrease in an allergy-causing protein, while those totally immersed in tap water had a 79 percent reduction in allergen level in the week after the washing. (Remember to wash your cat's face as well because there are lots of sebum-producing glands in the head area.)

bedroom. Wash your face, hands, and arms, too. Do not touch your face, especially your eyes, until after you have done so.

### Topical Products

Some topical products work to neutralize allergens on the skin and fur, and cats often prefer them to baths. However, the data on these products conflict with regard to their real effectiveness. Some are designed to be sprayed on; others are applied with a cloth to the fur. (Allerpet/C is one product that can be applied with a damp cloth.) Some products require daily application; others can be used less often. None have immediate effect. Pay special attention to spots that your cat licks most often. During dry spells, spray a bit of Allerpet or a similar substance on her coat to keep the dander from lifting off it and circulating throughout the house.

Nature's Miracle also produces Nature's Miracle Dander Remover and Deodorizer, Allerpet Allergy Relief, and Outright Allergy Relief. These nontoxic, nonstaining liquids are applied topically to your cat; just rub in and wipe off to clean away dander and soften her skin so that less dander is produced.

Another excellent product is the British-made Petal Cleanse/C for cats. It is a clear, colorless liquid with moisturizers that removes the dander and other allergens from the coat and encapsulates them. The moisturizers condition the coat and skin to further reduce the amount of hair and dander shed.

### Parasite Control

Skin parasites can cause itching and consequent scratching. When a cat scratches, dander flies and the skin becomes more irritated, and then even more dander is produced. The answer is simple—prevent fleas, ticks, and mites from infesting your cat in the first place.

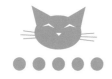

When a cat scratches too much, she produces more allergy-provoking dander. To reduce scratching, you'll have to control parasites.

Nowadays, there is no excuse for your cat not to be on an antiflea and tick program. Flea preventives come in two basic kinds: adulticides, which, as the name suggests, kill adult fleas on contact, and insect growth regulators (IGRs) such as Nylar, which stop little fleas from growing up into big ones and so halt the flea life cycle. IGRs don't kill adult fleas, though. Total prevention is usually the best plan.

### Neuter

Spayed and castrated cats have fewer hormonal swings and therefore tend to shed less and produce less sebum. This is especially true for male cats.

### Dietary Care

A poor diet or one that contains ingredients to which a cat is allergic can cause her to have skin problems. (That's how cats express *their* allergies rather than sneezing.) Add fatty acids to her diet to help keep her skin in top shape. Omega-3 and -6 fatty acids help the skin retain moisture, which can reduce shedding. Another product I use frequently is Mrs. Allen's Shed-Stop, a natural liquid dietary supplement with sunflower oil, vitamins, and anti-oxidants. Of course, it won't help with normal shedding, but it may work for cats who have a dietary deficiency. -

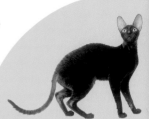

If it makes you feel any better, cats suffer allergies, too. It is estimated that 15 percent of cats in the US are allergic to one or more things. Your cat may be allergic to you!

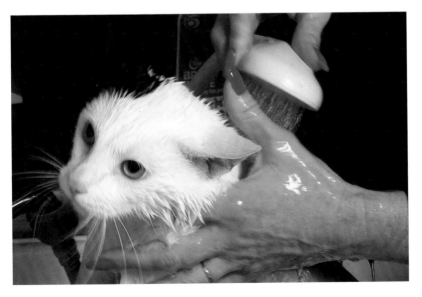

*Frequently bathing your cat could reduce the shedding of allergy-irritating proteins.*

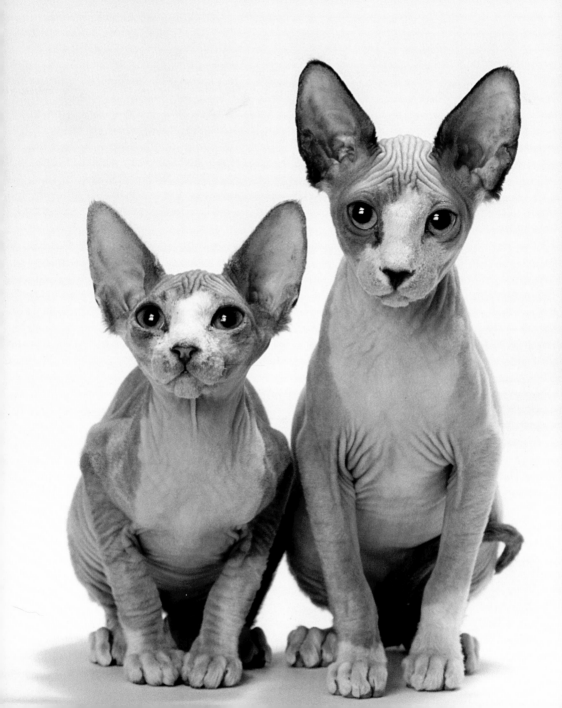

# Hypoallergenic Cats:
# FACT or FICTION?

While there is no such thing (yet) as a truly hypoallergenic cat, a number of breeds seem to have fewer allergy-producing effects on certain people than others. However, please remember that this is not a guarantee and that there are more substantial differences among individual cats than between any one breed and another. If you do decide to choose a cat belonging to one of these breeds, see if you can spend some time with the animal before bringing her home. And remember that some allergies take months to build up to the point at which symptoms develop.

There is nothing magical about so-called hypoallergenic cat breeds. They are simply breeds that in general and to varying degrees produce fewer allergens than run-of-the mill cats. They are not special in any other way. Remember that the prefix "hypo" does not mean "zero." It means "low." For people who are extremely allergic, "low" may well be too high. And while certain breeds of cat do seem to produce fewer allergens, other factors should also be taken into consideration. For example, males produce more allergens than females, unneutered males produce more allergens than neutered males, and for some reason, dark cats produce more allergens than light-colored ones!

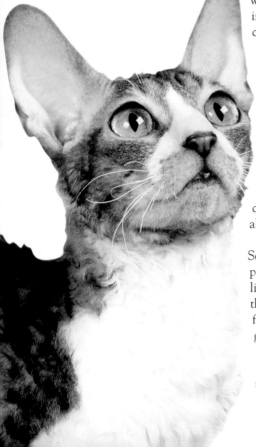

*Hypoallergenic cat breeds, like the Cornish Rex, are simply breeds that produce fewer allergens than regular cats.*

Hypoallergenic cats can be found in the same places regular cats are found—from high-priced breeders to low-cost animal shelters. Your brother-in-law may have one. One may wander in from the street. Some of these animals, including the Javanese and Balinese, are rare and as a consequence difficult to find.

However, breeders of all cat breeds may be found through the Fanciers Breeder Referral List at www.breedlist.com.

## DESIGNER CATS

Perhaps the ultimate answer for wannabe sneeze-free cat owners lies in technology. While no "natural" cat breed is truly hypoallergenic, a California biotechnology company, Allerca, has recently started taking orders for a hypoallergenic cat who they "designed" for pet lovers prone to allergies.

Their first hypoallergenic felines were born in September 2006. Unlike other companies that proposed the use of genetic engineering technologies like "gene silencing," Allerca bred its allergy-free cats the natural way. Thousands were tested in the search for the 1 cat in 50,000 who lacked the allergy-causing glycoprotein Fel d1. These animals were bred together until a strain of kittens without the Fel d1 protein was born. Although time consuming, this selective breeding program has a low potential for

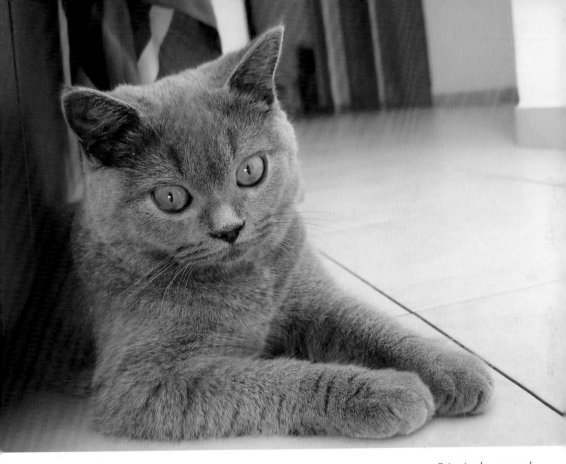

damaging side effects such as would occur with genetic modification (gene-silencing techniques that modify DNA).

Allerca president Simon Brodie says that he ultimately hopes to sell 200,000 of these cats annually in the United States. For obvious reasons, they will be neutered before sale. Because the target market for these animals is the allergic cat lover, it is believed that their sale will not hurt the adoption efforts of shelters.

The first breed of hypoallergenic cat will be the British Shorthair, which is friendly, affectionate, and playful. Even this breed, however, is not allergy-free. It simply produces much less allergens, Brodie explains. "It's like hypoallergenic makeup. The allergens are still there but in very small amounts that don't trigger allergic reactions." The British Shorthair is only the beginning, however. New examples are derived from the super gentle Ragamuffin breed. And what do the experts say about all this?

*Scientists have recently developed a cat that doesn't produce the allergy-causing protein Fel d1, which means they won't provoke allergic reactions in humans. The first breed available will be a British Shorthair.*

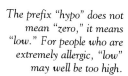

*The prefix "hypo" does not mean "zero," it means "low." For people who are extremely allergic, "low" may well be too high.*

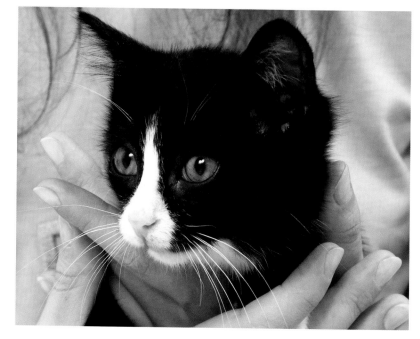

Approximately 2-15 percent of people are allergic to cats, and about a third of them have a cat in their home.

"I have my doubts that this is going to work," says David Rosenstreich, MD, Director of Allergy and Immunology at Albert Einstein School of Medicine in New York. "Fel d1 is the major protein to which patients are allergic, but cats produce other proteins that people are allergic to. Getting rid of Fel d1 will not create a completely nonallergenic cat." In addition,

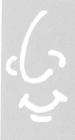

## Designer Dogs, too?

If you are a dog lover as well as a cat fancier, you should know that the same things that apply to cats also apply to dogs: There are no truly sneeze-free breeds for an extremely allergic person. However, there are several breeds that shed much less and thus are more "hypoallergenic." These include hairless breeds like the American Hairless Terrier and Mexican Hairless or Xoloitzcuintli; curly-coated breeds like Poodles (all varieties); the Bichon Frise; the Puli; terriers like Schnauzers (all varieties), the Bedlington Terrier, the Soft-Coated Wheaten Terrier, and the Kerry Blue Terrier; and single-coated breeds like the Basenji, Italian Greyhound, Maltese, Coton de Tulear, and Chihuahua.

there are some concerns that the gene producing the allergen may play a crucial role in some other part of the cat's metabolism, perhaps affecting the immune system.

Many facts about the new allergen-free cat will remain unknown for years. Dr. Gailen Marshall, Director of Clinical Immunology and Allergy at the University of Mississippi Medical Center, adds, "I'm not sure I like the idea of genetically manipulated cats, but I'll keep an open mind to it....it could be problematic over time. The allergen protein is very stable; it lives for long periods. This cat will still have dander, still groom itself, still have a kitty litter box. That cumulative amount could become an allergy issue—it's simply delayed rather than eliminated."

With all these caveats in mind, why not keep it simple. Let's take a look at some of the more well-known hypoallergenic breeds already available in nature (Chapter 4).

### Did You Know?

A hypoallergenic cat breed has recently been developed by scientists. Bred to not provoke an allergic reaction in humans, this designer cat enables many pet lovers with cat allergy to own and handle one.

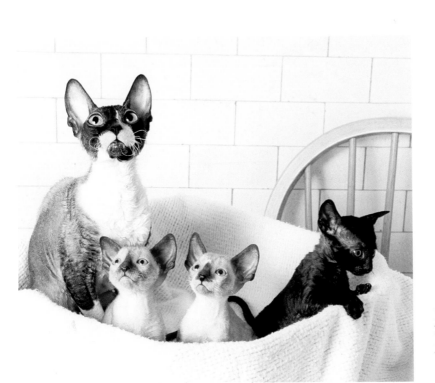

*Hypoallergenic cats can be found in the same places regular cats are found— from high-priced breeders to low-cost animal shelters.*

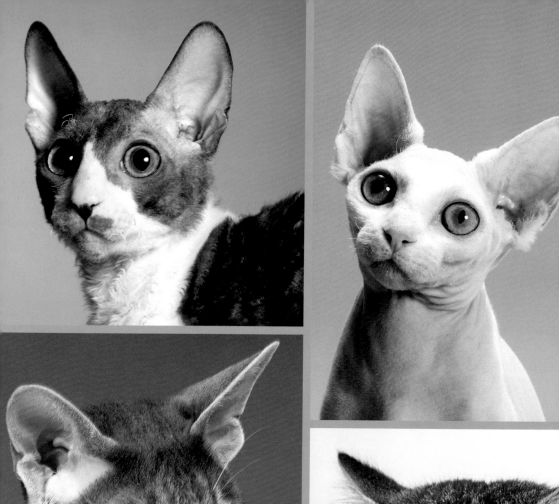
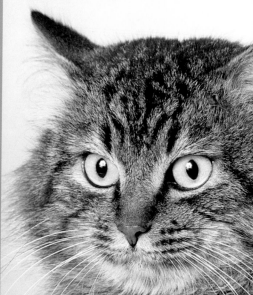
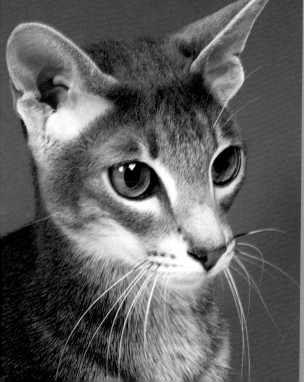

# Meet the
# BREEDS

In this section, we're going to take a look at some of the most hypoallergenic breeds. But whether or not a cat is hypoallergenic cannot be your only consideration in choosing a particular breed. The breed's temperament, activity level, habits, and other factors should be equally important factors in your decision. Always remember that every cat is an individual. With that in mind, please consider the *Vital Statistics* sections as general guidelines, not facts carved in stone. Aside from general characteristics, you will notice some health problems listed for most breeds as well. That does not mean that your cat is likely to get all (or even any) of them. It merely means that these problems have been noted in the breed.

It is very important to look beyond hypoallergenic qualities when looking for that "perfect cat." Read the breed profiles carefully and see if the named cat matches your needs. It's always best to find out these things before you get the cat—not after.

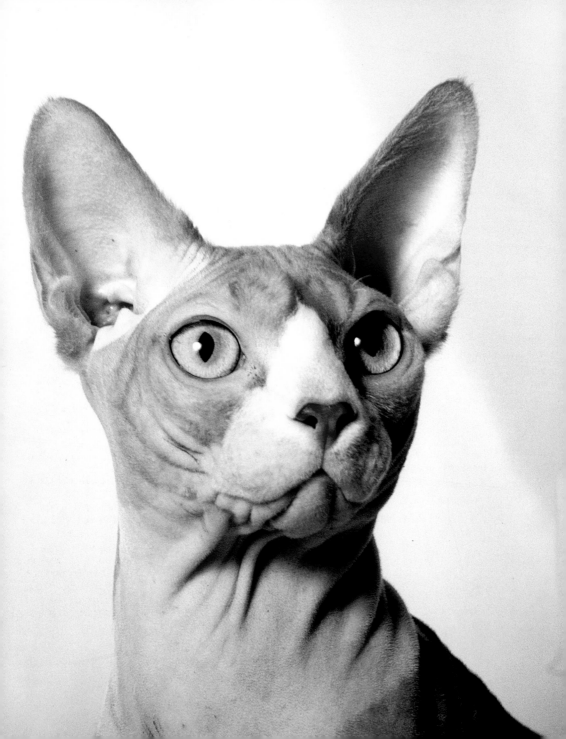

# SPHYNX

The first Sphynx cat was a fluke of nature; she was hairless. And while hairless dogs have been around for many centuries, the hairless cat is a comparative newcomer to the cat world (as far as we know, anyway). Interestingly, hairless cats have been reported in Latin America since the 1830s—the same place that hairless dogs come from.

## History

While hairless cats have been recorded periodically, the first recorded example of the cat subsequently known as the Sphynx appeared in Toronto, Canada, in 1966, thus making it the only natural Canadian breed of cat. They were first called "Moonstones" or "Canadian Hairless." The name "Sphynx" was given to the breed in the early 1970s by David Mare, a member of the Board of Directors of the Cat Fanciers' Association (CFA). Mare subsequently went on to breed them himself.

In studying the breed, Canadian geneticists and breeders discovered that the gene responsible for the hairlessness was an autosomal recessive trait. In other words, if you breed two hairless cats, all of their kittens will be hairless as well. If you breed a hairless cat with a normally coated cat, the kittens will appear normal but will carry the gene for hairlessness. If a kitten who carries the hairless gene is bred to a hairless cat, some of the kittens will probably be hairless. Although several generations of hairless cats were bred, breeders were unable to establish a stable body type and conformation for the line, so its registration was revoked.

The current version of the Sphynx dates back to 1975, when Wadena, Minnesota, farmers Milt and Ethylyn Pearson discovered a hairless kitten in a litter born to their apparently normal farm cat, a brown tabby named Jezabelle. The kitten was given the entirely appropriate name of Epidermis. Another such kitten, Dermis, was born the following year to the same mother. Both were sold to an Oregon cat breeder, Kim Mueske, who began

Hypoallergenic cats are animals that the breeder believes will produce fewer allergens than other cats. However, there are no guidelines, legal or otherwise, that determine to what degree this is true. If you have pet allergies, consult with your doctor before bringing home a cat.

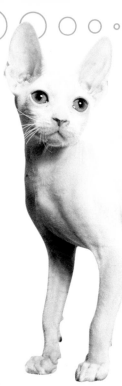

to develop the breed (with occasional outcrosses to the Cornish Rex, another hypoallergenic breed).

Another foundation cat for the breed was identified by Canadian Shirley Smith, a breeder of Siamese in the late 1970s and early 1980s. She discovered three hairless cats derived from three separate litters of a single black and white domestic cat bred to different males. The eldest kitten, Bambi, was in terrible shape. His left eye had been punctured in three places, and his genitalia were so badly mutilated that everything had to be removed. Still, he lived to be 19 years old. While he never (obviously) produced any kittens of his own, his appearance caught the attention of cat fanciers. Bambi's mother later produced two hairless female kittens out of two different males in 1979 and 1980. These two, Paloma and Punkie, were sent to Dr. Hugo Hernandez in Holland. Punkie was later bred to a white Devon Rex male, Curare van Jetrophin, a breeding that produced a litter of five kittens. Today, many Sphynx pedigrees go back to those two.

*The first officially documented example of the cat subsequently known as the Sphynx appeared in Toronto, Canada, in 1966.*

To keep the line, cat breeders in both Europe and North America have bred the Sphynx to normally coated cats and then back to hairless for more than 30 years. It's important to keep breeding back to normal animals so that a larger gene pool will be available and the resulting kittens will be healthy and vigorous. However, the breed's registration is currently "closed" in the United States, meaning that no further outcrosses are permitted; this is done to stabilize the qualities of the breed. Time will tell if the gene pool has been expanded sufficiently to prevent health problems.

So far, despite its strange appearance, the Sphynx breed is robust and appears to have very few health issues or genetic problems. In fact, you tend to get more health problems when you do outcross to the "general population." The breed's life span is that of a normal cat—15 years or longer. In fact, the oldest cat on record was a Sphynx named Grandpa Rex's Allen, who was estimated to have been 32 years of age when he finally passed away in 1998.

Grandpa belonged to Jacob Parry of Austin, Texas, who adopted him from a humane shelter in 1970. Parry, a retired plumber, along with his wife, Judy, had adopted over 400 cats. Grandpa was reputedly very fond of broccoli, which may or may not have accounted for his extreme longevity. He also drank coffee (Folger's). In addition, Grandpa had a special fondness for pink and enjoyed wearing pink sweaters to keep him warm and cozy. However, he would pull yellow or blue sweaters off.

Grandpa Rex's Allen was selected as the 1999 Cat of the Year in the debut issue of *Cats & Kittens* magazine. Of course, the award had to be given posthumously, but it was still well deserved. One might be tempted to wonder how Grandpa's precise age was obtained, but there's more to the story. Parry had a vague idea that there was something special about his hairless treasure, so he put up posters around the Austin area advertising his recently found hairless cat. He soon got a call from a Madame Sulinaberg of Paris (France, not Texas, although there is a Paris, Texas, too). She immediately identified the cat as "Pierre, mon chat!" For unclear reasons, said Madame agreed to let Parry keep the critter as long as he signed an agreement not to show the cat as a pedigreed animal. (She apparently did not like pedigree judges.) However, she eventually gave him the pedigree papers anyway, which revealed the cat's actual birth date to be February 1, 1964. The papers also declared his mother to have been a Sphynx named "Queen of France," while his father was a Devon Rex.

Parry kept his promise not to show his cat as a pedigreed beast, but he did start taking him around to shows as a house pet, although not until the cat reached the more mature years of his second decade. He eventually achieved the rank of Supreme Grand Master, given to him by the International Cat Association.

Because the gene pool for this breed is still very small, certain outcrosses are allowable. The CFA, for example, permits breeders to outcross the Sphynx with American Shorthairs or Domestic Shorthairs. Kittens born from these somewhat irregular unions are not likely to be top-quality show cats, but it's more important to increase the gene pool and keep the breed strong and vital. In addition, the hybrid Sphynx cats are often made available for adoption by breeders for little or no charge.

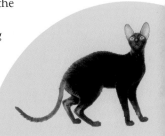

In 1902, a man named Shinick in Albuquerque, New Mexico, acquired two hairless littermates, Nellie and Dick, from local Pueblo Indians.

To be registered with the CFA, kittens born on or after December 31, 2010, may have only Sphynx parents.

## Appearance and Temperament

The highly intelligent Sphynx is a sturdy, medium-sized cat, with males substantially (up to 25 percent) larger than females. The chest is broad, almost to the point of being barrel chested. They have very large ears. The eyes usually conform to coat color, and all eye colors are acceptable in the breed.

The Sphynx breed looks as if it is *extremely* wrinkled, although it doesn't actually have any more wrinkles than any other cat—in other breeds, the wrinkles are covered by hair. (Kittens, however, seem to be more wrinkled than the adults.) All color patterns are allowed, except those that are determined by the placement of color on a single shaft of hair (shaded, cameo, smoke, chinchilla, ticked). It's odd to think of naked cats as having colors, but they are painted right there on the skin. Interestingly, exposure to sun will intensify all colors, but these cats can get sunburned.

Sphynx cats are curious and energetic, and they enjoy your undivided attention; in fact, they often perform tricks and antics to get it. They are great "starers," and many people regard their temperaments as nothing other than flirtatious. The French breed standard says that the Sphynx is part monkey, part cat, part child, and part dog. They are known to wag their tails like dogs when pleased, and they become extremely attached to their owners (and strangers, too, often leaping onto their laps or shoulders

*Although the Sphynx looks extremely wrinkled, it doesn't actually have any more wrinkles than any other cat—in other breeds, the wrinkles are covered by hair.*

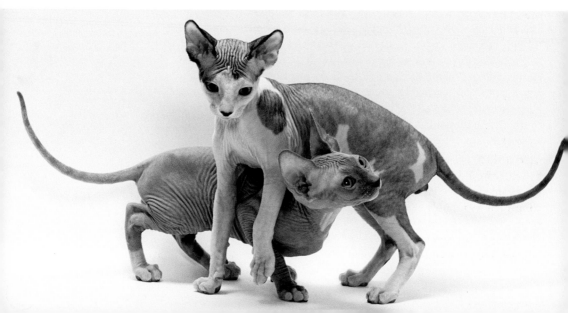

without waiting for an invitation). Many learn to play fetch, and in general, they enjoy interactive games with their humans. They do have a reputation, though, for being slightly clumsy for a cat, a trait attributed to their scarcity of whiskers.

One of the oddest things about this breed is the precocity of the kittens, who are said to open their eyes when they are only two or three days old. They are also adept at climbing out of their "cribs" when they are just three weeks old. At that age, they begin weaning and using the litter box.

Along with human company, Sphynx cats like the company of other cats and even dogs. (In fact, they often seem to demand a playmate.) Remember, however, that as an allergy sufferer, the more animals you have, the greater stress you're putting on your immune system.

A hairless animal like the Sphynx still produces allergens, but there is no coat for dander to cling to or hair to deposit all over the house. Actually, many Sphynx cats are not completely hairless and have a fine down on the body, which makes them feel, some say, "like a warm peach." Because they have no fur, they are quite warm to the touch. In addition, the Sphynx is apt to have hair on the nose, tail, and toes. The skin itself has a chamois or suede-like texture (rather nice once you get used to it).

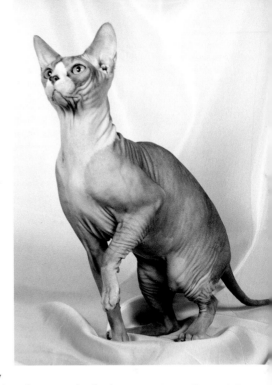

*Highly intelligent, Sphynx cats are curious, energetic, and bond closely to their owners.*

The greatest danger to these cats is that they suffer from the cold, as you might expect, which for them is anything below 70°F (21.1°C). In even colder weather, they may grow a bit of "fuzz." If it's cold for you, it's cold for them. (Some cats will consent to wear a sweater.) Not only have they no protection from the heat and cold, but their naked skin provides a feast for mosquitoes and other insects, and it is vulnerable to thorns and burrs. Remember that these cats don't have eyelashes or hairs in the ears to protect them, so they are vulnerable to eye tearing and dirt in the ears. Sphynx cats also seem to have poorer teeth than normally coated cats. (The same is true with hairless dogs.) The "hairless" gene is apparently connected with tooth health. Brushing the teeth frequently is very helpful in this regard.

The Sphynx benefits from bathing more than most cats because it removes the excess oils (and allergens) from the skin. Altered cats require bathing at least once every other week, but more frequent baths are even better. Unnuetered males (not a good idea for allergy sufferers) need to be bathed every other day or so. If you don't wash them, you'll end up with a brown, oily residue on the skin, which is far from pretty.

When bathing your Sphynx, use antibacterial antifungal soap designed especially for sensitive skin. With a hairless cat, baths are quick and so is the drying off process. However, if you're in a real hurry, you don't even have to put the cat under water; using gentle baby wipes also does an excellent job. And after all, your cat is your baby. Whether it's because of their unusual size or not, Sphynx ears seem to get unusually dirty and require frequent cleaning as well. It's also wise to clean out the fold of skin behind each claw, which seems to accumulate allergen-bearing secretions.

Remember, this breed is not allergy-proof. Sphynx cats produce dandruff directly on their skin, and even though they produce less of it than normally coated animals, they can still produce enough to trigger an allergic reaction.

The biggest downside to owning a Sphynx, from the point of view of many owners, is that some of them have terrible litter box manners. Some refuse to cover their leavings, while others just skip the whole litter box ordeal altogether. They also have a tremendous appetite, and as shown in the aforementioned case of Grandpa Rex's Allen, seem to prefer people food, including vegetables, and often steal them directly off the plate.

Because this breed is still quite rare, they are expensive, and breeders have long waiting lists. You can expect to bring a Sphynx kitten home when she is between 12 and 16 weeks old and is thoroughly immunized.

## Association Acceptance

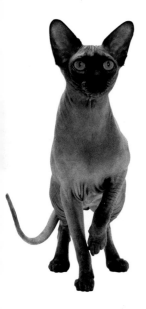

In the cat show world, the breed continued to gain popularity in the 1990s. It won acceptance into the American Cat Fanciers Association (ACFA) Championship class in 1994 and the Cat Fanciers' Association (CFA) Miscellaneous class in February 1998, and it is currently shown in the CFA for Championship class as well. There are now five major international breeder groups (International Sphynx Breeders and Fanciers Association [ISBFA], National Association of Sphynx and Rex [NASAR], Progressive Sphynx Alliance [PSA], Sphynx and Rex Association [SARA], Sphynx Cat Association [SCA]) that recognize the Sphynx as a breed. The Sphynx is accepted for championship by:

- American Association of Cat Enthusiasts (AACE)
- American Cat Association (ACA)

- American Cat Fanciers Association (ACFA)
- Canadian Cat Association (CCA)
- Cat Fanciers' Association (CFA)
- Cat Fanciers Federation (CFF)
- The International Cat Association (TICA)
- United Feline Organization (UFO)

## THE SPHYNX AT A GLANCE

**General Appearance:** Hairless or with peach-like fuzz. Medium build and size, with females smaller than males. The body is soft and warm to the touch. The texture of the skin should resemble a peach.

**Head:** Modified wedge, slightly longer than wide. Skull slightly rounded, nose straight with a slight stop where the nose meets the forehead.

**Cheeks:** Prominent but rounded.

**Muzzle:** Strong chin, whisker break with prominent whisker pads.

**Ears:** Quite large, broad at the base, open, upright when viewed from the front; the outer edge of the base of the ear should begin at eye level.

**Eyes:** Large and lemon shaped, coming to a definite point on each side. They should angle slightly upward and be set wide apart. Any color acceptable.

**Neck:** Medium in length, rounded, well muscled, slightly arched.

**Body:** Medium length, muscular, medium boned. Broad chest and rounded abdomen.

**Legs and Paws:** Legs medium in proportion to the body. Sturdy and well muscled. Oval paws, with five toes in front and four behind. Paw pads should be thick and cushiony.

**Tail:** Slender, whiplike, and flexible.

**Color:** Any.

**Faults:** Improper hair or coat. Frail appearance. Bowed front legs. Thin in the abdomen, rump, or chest. Should not resemble the Devon Rex, Cornish Rex, or Oriental body type.

**Disqualifications:** Kinked tail, structural abnormalities. Aggression.

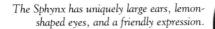

*The Sphynx has uniquely large ears, lemon-shaped eyes, and a friendly expression.*

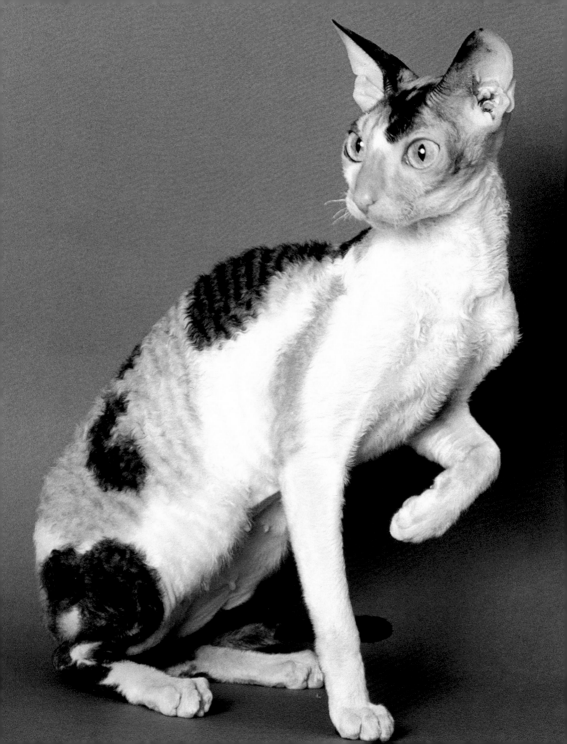

# CORNISH REX

The exotic Cornish Rex is an extremely affectionate and people-oriented breed. These playful cats are perfect pets for anyone who wants a fun and energetic companion to participate in daily family life. And the good news for allergy sufferers is that, compared to other cats, shedding is minimal.

## History

The first Cornish Rex cat was discovered on July 21, 1950, in Cornwall, England. In a normal litter of five kittens born to a tortoiseshell and white domestic cat named Serena appeared a curly-coated orange and white male, subsequently named Kallibunker by the litter owner, Nina Ennismore. Kallibunker was different from his littermates in many ways. Aside from the curly coat, he had big ears, a wedge-shaped head, and a long, racy, lithe body. Perhaps a foreign male was involved. (Because a litter of cats can have more than one father, it is perfectly possible that Kallibunker's parentage was not identical to that of his littermates.) However that may be, Kallibunker was backcrossed to Serena, and more curly-coated kittens appeared. (Incest is a common ploy of animal breeders when trying to produce a new line.) The breed arrived in the United States in 1957 in the form of LaMorna Cove, the first to produce kittens.

## Appearance and Temperament

The name "Cornish" comes from Cornwall, the area of England in which the breed first appeared, and "Rex" is derived from the curly-coated Astrex Rabbit. The Cornish Rex does have a soft, rabbit fur-like quality to her coat, although many compare the texture to lambswool, velvet, or silk. Partly due to the lack of guard hairs that impart the stiff quality most cats' or dogs' coats have, the hair becomes increasingly soft as the cat matures. This is because the coat consists only of the very soft "awn" hairs that form a tight wave lying close to the body, which is called "rexing." Whiskers are

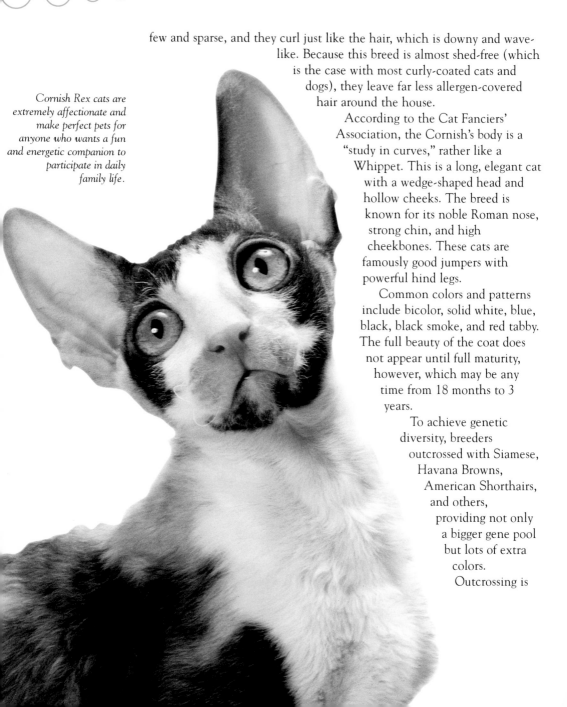

few and sparse, and they curl just like the hair, which is downy and wave-like. Because this breed is almost shed-free (which is the case with most curly-coated cats and dogs), they leave far less allergen-covered hair around the house.

*Cornish Rex cats are extremely affectionate and make perfect pets for anyone who wants a fun and energetic companion to participate in daily family life.*

According to the Cat Fanciers' Association, the Cornish's body is a "study in curves," rather like a Whippet. This is a long, elegant cat with a wedge-shaped head and hollow cheeks. The breed is known for its noble Roman nose, strong chin, and high cheekbones. These cats are famously good jumpers with powerful hind legs.

Common colors and patterns include bicolor, solid white, blue, black, black smoke, and red tabby. The full beauty of the coat does not appear until full maturity, however, which may be any time from 18 months to 3 years.

To achieve genetic diversity, breeders outcrossed with Siamese, Havana Browns, American Shorthairs, and others, providing not only a bigger gene pool but lots of extra colors. Outcrossing is no longer permitted, however. Also, because the breed's unusual hair type is caused by a recessive gene, you can only guarantee that a kitten will have the desirable coat type if two Cornish Rex cats are bred to each other. Some theorists maintain that the gene mutation responsible for the hair types was caused by radiation from a local tin mine, but there is no evidence to support this view; mutations have occurred for millions of years, with or without tin mines.

Generally, Cornish Rex cats are not difficult to care for. They usually require regular bathing because of the oily secretions that build up on their coats. This is true even for cats who don't have allergic owners. Don't follow the bath with a moisturizing rinse, because it can ruin the coat. An added benefit for allergy sufferers, Cornish Rex cats are very easy to bathe because soap penetrates the short fur easily, and it dries fast. This same quality, however, makes them very susceptible to cold, from which they must always be protected. And as is true of most hypoallergenic breeds, their ears can build up waxy secretions very quickly and so need frequent cleaning.

Generally hearty and long-lived, the Cornish Rex does have a powerful appetite, unlike the typical finicky feline. As a result, these cats can gain weight easily. Other health problems include hypothyroidism (low thyroid hormone levels resulting in a loss of curl to the hair, followed by hair loss) and hypotrichosis (hair loss resulting in permanent baldness by six months of age). However, most Cornish Rex cats are quite healthy and commonly live until age 18 or 20. They retain their playfulness into old age.

Very social and animated, these cats are usually quite easy to handle. They like to steal objects and then retrieve them, and they are excellent jumpers and climbers. They are not above jumping from the tops of doors onto visitors or the family dog, so be forewarned. In fact, this breed is excessively fond of canines. Not quiet lap cats, they prefer a home where they can exercise their relentless energy. Extremely active and playful, this breed seems to enjoy travel—unlike most cats. They also like to be petted and handled.

As with many pedigree breeds, pricing and availability varies with type, markings, and bloodlines. Breeders usually will make kittens available between 12 and 16 weeks. At 12 weeks, kittens have been properly inoculated and socialized and are able to adapt to a new environment. It is always advisable to keep such cats indoors, as well as to neuter them to help ensure a healthy, long, and joyful life.

**Did You Know?**

The name "Cornish" comes from Cornwall, the area of England in which the breed first appeared.

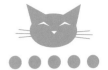

The Cornish Rex is a long, elegant cat known for its noble Roman nose, strong chin, and high cheekbones.

## Association Acceptance

The Cat Fanciers' Association (CFA) accepted the Cornish Rex as a breed in 1962.

The breed is currently accepted by the following associations:

- American Association of Cat Enthusiasts (AACE)
- American Cat Association (ACA)
- American Cat Fanciers Association (ACFA)
- Canadian Cat Association (CCA)
- Cat Fanciers' Association (CFA)
- Cat Fanciers Federation (CFF)
- The International Cat Association (TICA)
- United Feline Organization (UFO)

*Not quiet lap cats, Cornish Rex prefer a home where they can exercise their relentless energy. Commonly living until age 18 or 20, they retain their playfulness into old age.*

# THE CORNISH REX AT A GLANCE

**General Appearance:** Racy body type, and soft, wavy "marcelled" coat.

**Profile:** Distinctive. Two convex arcs form a curve. In fact, all contours of the cat are curvy.

**Head:** Egg-shaped, fairly small head, about one-third longer than wide. Rounded forehead. Roman nose. Strong whisker break.

**Neck:** Long and slender.

**Muzzle:** Narrowing slightly.

**Ears:** Larger the better. Full at the base. Set high on the head.

**Nose:** Roman, one-third the length of the head.

**Cheeks:** High, prominent, well-chiseled cheekbones.

**Chin:** Strong, well developed.

**Body:** Small to medium. Males somewhat larger than females. Long and slender, not tubular. Chest deep but not broad. Arched back.

**Legs:** Long and slender. "Stands high." This is a distinguishing characteristic.

**Paws:** Dainty, slightly oval. Five toes in front and four in back.

**Tail:** Long, slender, flexible, and tapering.

**Coat:** Short, silky, soft, fairly dense. Tight marcel wave.

**Colors:** Wide variety in many patterns, including: solid, shaded, smoke, tabby, bicolor, particolor, and pointed.

**Faults:** Sparse coat or bare spots.

**Disqualifications:** Kinked tail, incorrect number of toes. Lameness or any sign of poor health. Outcrosses are not permitted in this breed.

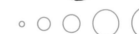

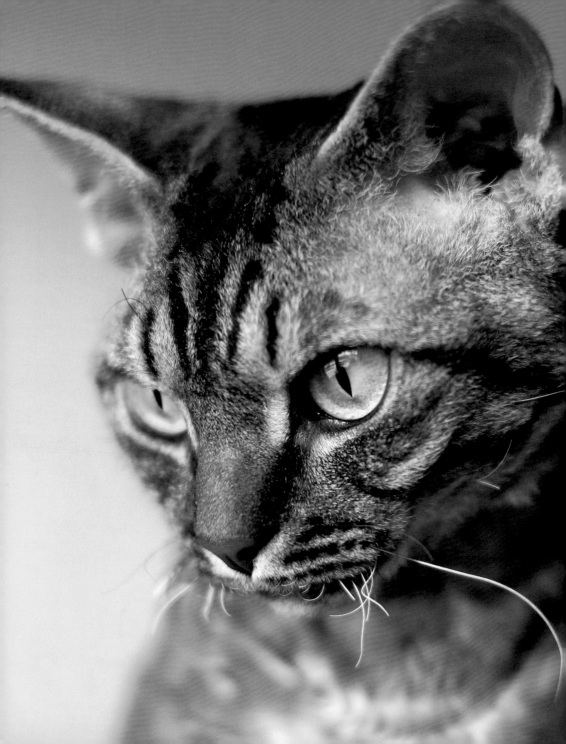

# DEVON REX

The Devon Rex is similar in appearance to the Cornish Rex, although the two are not closely related. These low-maintenance, wash-and-wear companions are highly active, playful, and like to be involved in everything. Unusual pixie-like features highlight the perky personality, high intelligence, and friendliness for which these cats are known and desired.

## History

The Devon was imported into the United States in 1968. The "founding father" of the breed, however, was born to a litter in Devonshire, England in 1959. He was actually the offspring of a feral animal who mated with a calico female. One of the kittens from this mating was a brown-black male that the owner, Beryl Cox, named Kirlee. Even today, Kirlee's looks remain the standard of perfection.

When the first Devons were bred, the mating initially did not produce any curly-coated kittens. The problem turned out to be that while Kirlee was bred to other Cornish curly-coated cats, the curls were caused by two different mutations, a fact not discovered until later. Kirlee's curl mutation was late gene II Rex, while the other mutation was gene I Rex. A few cats, both Devon and Cornish, who carry the double Rex heritage, still exist. Kirlee eventually sired ten Rex Gen II litters before he was retired and neutered. He lived the remainder of his life as a pet until he died in 1970, falling victim to a street accident.

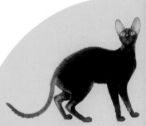

A rare and select breed known for its odd yet striking appearance, the Devon Rex began emerging in England during the 1960s and was imported into the US in 1968.

## Appearance and Temperament

Devons are smaller than Cornish, with round heads, large round eyes, and big ears that are seemingly disproportionate to the rest of their bodies. They often have less and shorter fur than their Cornish counterparts and a more flowing, less marcelled appearance. An even flow of loose curls is

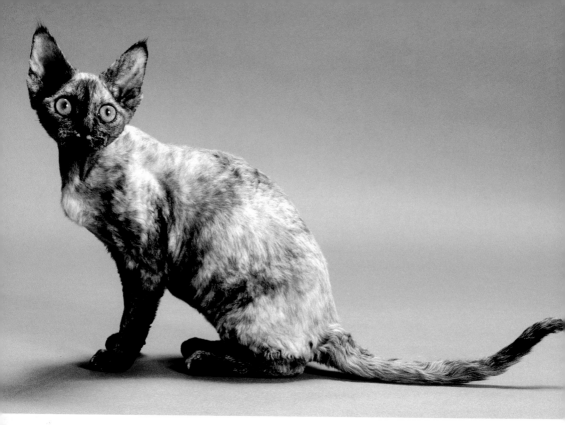

*Although the Devon Rex is somewhat similar in appearance to the Cornish Rex, the two breeds are not closely related.*

considered ideal for the show ring. The Devon has a birth coat that is substantially different from her adult one, but it will shed out at about eight weeks of age in favor of a thicker, more substantial coat. Some of these cats can look rather bald, although bare patches are a fault in the show ring. Like the Cornish, this breed sheds very little, which makes it more acceptable to people with allergies.

Unlike the Cornish coat, which lacks guard hairs, the Devon coat has all three hair types (guard, awn, and down), although the guard hairs are fragile and often stunted. Many lack whiskers completely; others have wrinkled or crinkled ones. The same is true of the eyebrows. Because the coat lacks good insulation, these animals need to be kept warm. They are "heat seekers" who try to get as close to their owners as possible.

The coat needs natural oils dispersed down each hair shaft to lie correctly and wave. Oils also collect between the paw pads and must be cleaned out. Devons can be bathed by a simple wipe down with a damp washcloth and don't require full baths the way the Sphynx and Cornish

Rex do. However, baths won't hurt, and allergy sufferers should consider bathing their cat about once a week.

Extremely social and animated, Devons require your attention and will entertain you with their antics and inquisitive nature. Many have a charming elfin expression (partly due to the upturned nose), which is unlike that of any other cat. Like the Cornish Rex, they are famously good jumpers but often like best to ride around on your shoulders. They make wonderful companions.

Health problems in the breed include congenital patellar subluxation, hypothyroidism (most cats are more likely to be hyperthyroidistic), hip dysplasia, and spasticity (a neurological condition in which the cat is unable to chew and swallow properly).

Currently, outcrossing is permitted with the American or British Shorthair. However, kittens born on or after May 1, 2013, may have only Devon Rex parents.

## Association Acceptance

The breed was accepted by the American Cat Fanciers Association (ACFA) in 1972 and by the International Cat Association (TICA) in 1972 (the year that the organization was formed.). Because the gene pool is

The Devon's unusual pixie-like features highlight the perky personality, high intelligence, and friendliness for which the breed is known and desired.

*Low-maintenance, wash-and-wear companions, Devon Rex cats are highly active, playful, and like to be involved in everything.*

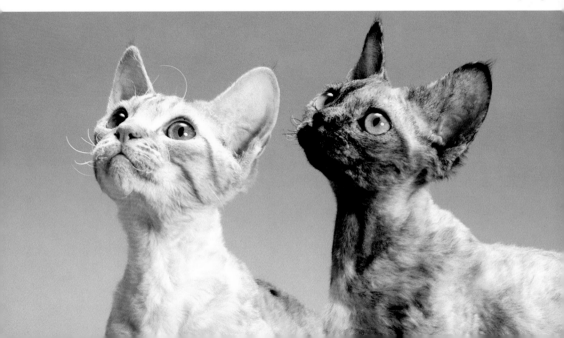

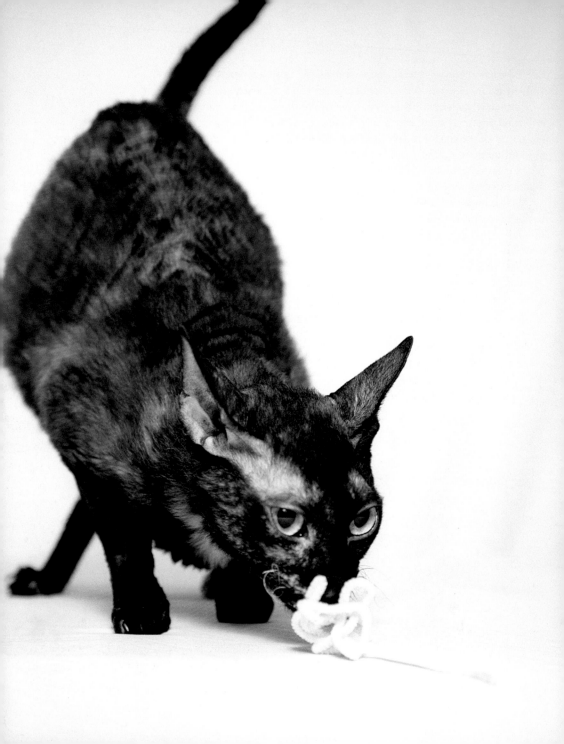

still very small, many breeders continue to outcross to other breeds (not the Cornish Rex, though, whose coat is caused by a different mutation).

The breed is accepted by the following associations:

- American Association of Cat Enthusiasts (AACE)
- American Cat Association (ACA)
- American Cat Fanciers Association (ACFA)
- Canadian Cat Association (CCA)
- Cat Fanciers' Association (CFA)
- Cat Fanciers Federation (CFF)
- The International Cat Association (TICA)
- Traditional Cat Association, Inc. (TCA)
- United Feline Organization (UFO)

Extremely social and animated, Devons require your attention and will entertain you with their antics and inquisitive nature.

## THE DEVON REX AT A GLANCE

**General Appearance:** Pixie-like face, large eyes, short muzzle, prominent cheekbones, very large, low-set ears. Soft, wavy fur.

**Head:** Modified wedge, slightly longer than broad. Strongly marked stop.

**Muzzle:** Short, well developed. Prominent whisker pads.

**Chin:** Strong, well developed.

**Neck:** Medium and slender.

**Eyes:** Wide set, large, oval, sloping toward the outer edges of the ears. Any color acceptable.

**Ears:** Very large, low set, wide at the base, tapering to rounded tops.

**Body:** Muscular, hard, broad in the chest. Hind legs somewhat longer than front legs. Males are larger.

**Legs and Paws:** Legs slender and long. Feet oval and small, with five toes in front and four behind.

**Coat:** Hair densest on the back, sides, tail, legs, and ears. Top of the head, chest, and abdomen may have less dense hair. Hair is soft, fine, and full bodied.

**Faults:** Narrow, long, round, or domestic-type head, extremely short muzzle, misaligned bite, small, high-set ears, bare patches.

**Disqualifications:** Extensive baldness, kinked or abnormal tail, incorrect number of toes, crossed eyes, weak hind legs.

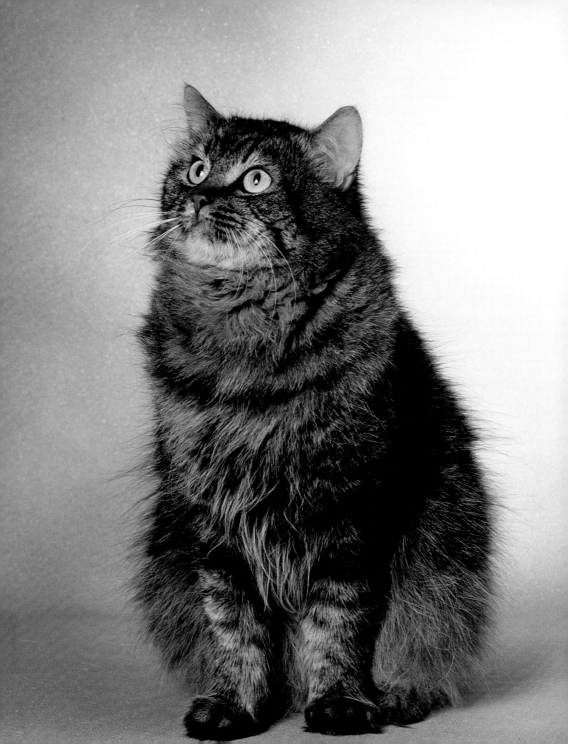

# The
# SIBERIAN CAT

Although they have been around for a very long time, the Siberian is somewhat rare in the United States, and most breeders have long waiting lists for this delightful, dutiful, almost "dog-like" cat who will greet you at the door and follow you around the house. They make excellent family pets, and despite their somewhat long, plush coats, they are a good choice for prospective owners who suffer from allergies.

## History

The very beautiful Siberian cat is one of the ancient cat breeds, with a history stretching back more than 1,000 years. As the name suggests, this breed originated in Russia and is sometimes called the Russian Forest Cat. The Siberian is considered a "natural" cat breed, one that developed on its own in a local area, rather than one encouraged by human beings in the way that the Sphynx and Rex breeds were developed. The first Siberian cats were imported to the United States in 1990 after the dissolution of the USSR.

## Appearance and Temperament

Unlike other cats considered to be hypoallergenic, the Siberian has a semi-long and luxuriant (but nonmatting) coat. The breed comes in all colors (color patterns are the same as in Persians), although because of the extreme rarity of the breed in the United States, not all colors are easily found. The most common coloration is a brown mackerel tabby, some with white and some without.

This is a very large cat, comparable in size to the Maine Coon. It's a slow-maturing breed that doesn't reach full adulthood until it is five years

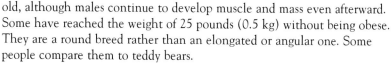 

A natural breed and the national cat of Russia, the Siberian has been around for at least 1000 years.

The Siberian is one of the few long-haired breeds considered to be hypoallergenic.

old, although males continue to develop muscle and mass even afterward. Some have reached the weight of 25 pounds (0.5 kg) without being obese. They are a round breed rather than an elongated or angular one. Some people compare them to teddy bears.

The Siberian has a sweet facial expression. The eyes are large, round, and usually yellow-green. The ears are wide at the base, with Lynx tipping. Tipped ears are highly desirable, and lots of soft hair on the ears is a requirement.

Of special interest to allergy sufferers are the hypoallergenic qualities of the Siberian's fur, a fact discovered in 1995 by breeder Lynda Nelson of Kravchenko Siberians.

This breed apparently produces very little dander and sheds very little. However, these fluffy cats do shed out twice a year, and while this may sound like a nightmare for allergy sufferers, Siberians appear to have lower-than-average enzyme levels in their saliva. Usually, when a cat cleans herself, the offending protein dries on the fur, leaving dander. However, some breeders claim that the Siberian is void of the Fel d1 protein, thereby producing no dander. Therefore, if the allergic party suffers from the IgE late trigger antibody reaction, their chances of compatibility with a Siberian are lowered as a result. Another theory is that because of the tight, thick undercoat and oily top coat, the skin stays well hydrated, thereby reducing dander production and distribution. This seems more likely to me. Interestingly, it has also been proven that hair length has no bearing on the severity of the symptoms that the allergy sufferer will have. Some estimate that about 75 percent of cat allergy sufferers show no reaction to this breed.

Siberians are affectionate, playful, and agile, although they sometimes exhibit a bit of good-natured zaniness. Showing great loyalty to their families, many of them bond strongly and are apt to spend lots of time with their loved ones; some even come when they are called. Lots of them like to play fetch, too. They are superb jumpers and like to play with other cats, dogs, and even children. Some appear to take on a protective role toward the youngest members of the family, sleeping at the foot of the bed and "guarding" them. However, in other respects they are really just like every other cat—thinking of themselves first and foremost.

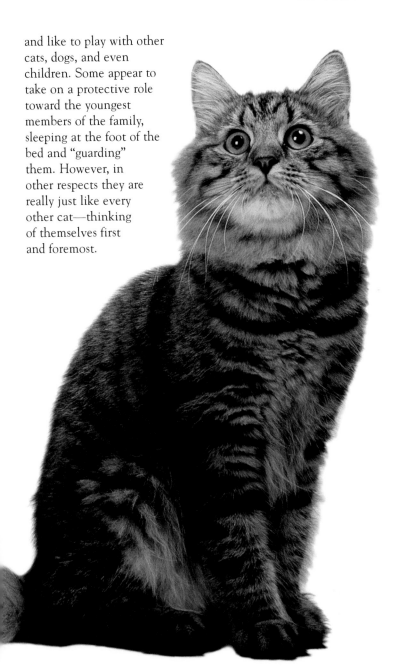

*The very beautiful Siberian is a delightful, dutiful, almost "dog-like" cat who will greet you at the door and follow you around the house.*

## Did You Know?

A large cat weighing up to 25 lbs, Siberians are affectionate, playful, and agile, although they sometimes exhibit a bit of good-natured zaniness.

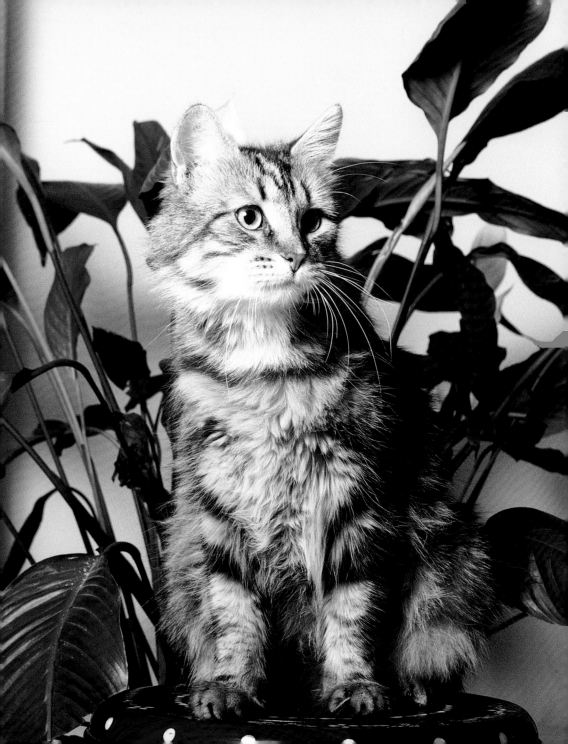

The Siberian is generally a very hearty, healthy breed, although there have been a few cases of umbilical hernia (which can be repaired by surgery).

No outcrosses are permitted.

## Association Acceptance

The Siberian is accepted in the provisional cats class by the Cat Fanciers' Association (CFA), and the breed is accepted for championship by the following North American cat associations:

- American Association of Cat Enthusiasts (AACE)
- American Cat Association (ACA)
- American Cat Fanciers Association (ACFA)
- Cat Fanciers Federation (CFF)
- National Cat Fanciers' Association (NCFA)
- The International Cat Association (TICA)
- United Feline Organization (UFO)

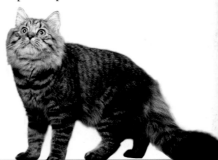

# THE SIBERIAN AT A GLANCE

**General Appearance:** Medium large, powerful, but with a sweet facial expression.

**Head:** Modified wedge, with rounded contours. Whiskers are strong. Top of the head is flat. Head should be set off by a ruff.

**Muzzle:** Full and slightly rounded.

**Ears:** Medium wide at the base, rounded tips with Lynx tipping.

**Eyes:** Large, round, wide set.

**Body:** Substantial, back medium in length, slightly curved.

**Legs and Paws:** Thick and dense, big feet. Toe tufts desirable.

**Tail:** Medium, somewhat shorter than the length of the body.

**Coat:** Plush, of medium length. A tight undercoat.

**Faults:** Lack of substance, straight profile, almond-shaped eyes, thin legs.

**Disqualifications:** Kinked tail, incorrect number of toes.

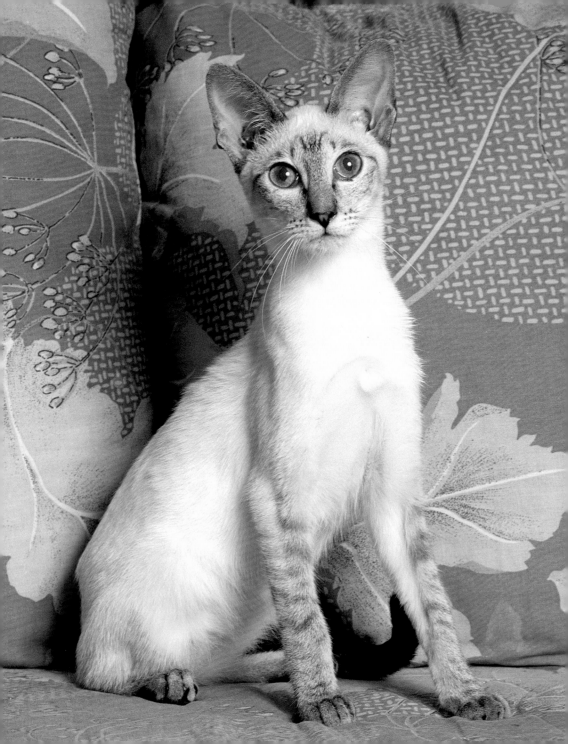

# BALINESE

Balinese were once called the "long-haired Siamese" and do resemble them, although they are thankfully somewhat less vocal and have a softer voice. Lovers of the breed claim that they speak only when they have something to say. With their ermine coats and sparkling sapphire eyes, they are quite alluring and present a rather regal bearing. Yet they are also clowns at heart. Affectionate, curious, and demonstrative, these elegant Oriental felines captivate any animal lover. This breed and its cousin, the Javanese, are difficult to find—especially if you live in the middle of the US. You will have better luck if you live on either of the two coasts, although some breeders are willing to ship their kittens.

## History

Despite their names, Balinese do not come from Bali. The name was given to them by breeder-judge Helen Smith of Long Island, New York, who thought they were as graceful as Balinese dancers.

The breed may have developed as a spontaneous or natural mutation, although this is debated. Most believe that they were a spontaneous mutation of the Siamese cat in the early 1900s. Because their coat types were at first considered undesirable, individuals possessing Balinese gave them away to pet homes. Concerted breeding efforts did not begin until the 1940s. In many ways, the breeding of Balinese is difficult and somewhat unrewarding because they must be bred back to the Siamese regularly to preserve type. Of course, the short-haired kittens resulting from this breeding will not be able to be shown as Balinese, although they do carry the long-haired gene for future generations.

The Balinese cat was given its name because the breed was considered to have the grace and beauty of a Balinese dancer.

## Appearance and Temperament

Balinese are lithe, energetic cats with striking, deep blue eyes. This is a colorpoint breed, which generally has darker colors on the face, ears, and extremities. It comes in chocolate, blue, lilac, seal, lynx, and particolor,

Balinese are very active, affectionate cats—and they even get along with dogs.

although not all colors are accepted by all cat registries. The CFA accepts only the traditional points of the Siamese: seal, chocolate, blue, and lilac. The breed has a fine, silky, single coat that lies close to the body, not standing out in the way that the coat of most long-haired breeds does. Balinese are often described as svelte, dainty cats with long, tapering body lines. Although long and slim, they are very lithe and muscular. Their most distinctive feature is a long, luxuriously plumed tail.

These loving cats demand attention and are quite fond of riding on their owners' shoulders, fetching toys, and generally satisfying their healthy curiosity. They are very active and get along quite well with dogs.

As with the other hypoallergenic breeds, Balinese produce significantly less Fel d1 than most other cats, thus provoking less allergic reactions. As an additional advantage, grooming is easy because the long, single coat does not mat.

Although healthy overall, some Balinese have problems with gingivitis and cardiomyopathy, a heart disease.

This breed may be outcrossed to the Siamese.

## Association Acceptance

The Balinese is accepted for championship by the following cat associations:

- American Association of Cat Enthusiasts (AACE)
- American Cat Association (ACA)
- American Cat Fanciers Association (ACFA)
- Canadian Cat Association (CCA)
- Cat Fanciers' Association (CFA)
- Cat Fanciers Federation (CFF)
- National Cat Fanciers' Association (NCFA)
- The International Cat Association (TICA)
- Traditional Cat Association (TCA)
- United Feline Organization (UFO)

*Balinese are lithe, energetic cats with striking, deep blue eyes.*

# THE BALINESE AT A GLANCE

The breed description here applies to the modern Balinese. However, some breeders are harking back to the more traditional Balinese (sometimes called the "apple-headed" Balinese) who only fell out of favor during the 1950s and 1960s but have lately been making something of resurgence. These animals are considerably heavier and have a more robust body than the modern Balinese. They also have longer hair (2 inches (5.1 cm) and more) over the entire body, not just on the tail. Today, only modern Balinese are seen at cat shows.

**General Appearance:** Long tubular body with a fine silky coat. Tail plume.

**Head:** Tapering wedge. No less than the width of an eye between the eyes. Flat skull, no bulge over the eyes.

**Ears:** Very large, pointed. Wide at the base.

**Eyes:** Almond shaped, medium size. Slanted toward the nose, uncrossed.

**Nose:** Long and straight.

**Muzzle:** Wedge shaped, fine.

**Chin and Jaw:** Medium size.

**Neck:** Long and slender.

**Body:** Graceful, medium size. Males may be larger than females.

**Legs:** Long and slim. Hind legs higher than front.

**Paws:** Small and dainty. Five toes in front, four in back.

**Tail:** Long, tapering.

**Coat:** Medium length, fine, silky. Longest on the tail. No downy undercoat.

**Color:** Seal point (dark brown), chocolate point (warm brown), blue point (slate), and lilac (rose-gray) point.

**Faults:** Lack of pigment in the nose leather or paw pads. Crossed eyes.

**Disqualifications:** Evidence of illness. Weak hind legs. Malocclusion. Visible kink in the tail. Eye color other than blue. Definite double coat.

*The Balinese's most distinctive feature is a long, luxuriously plumed tail.*

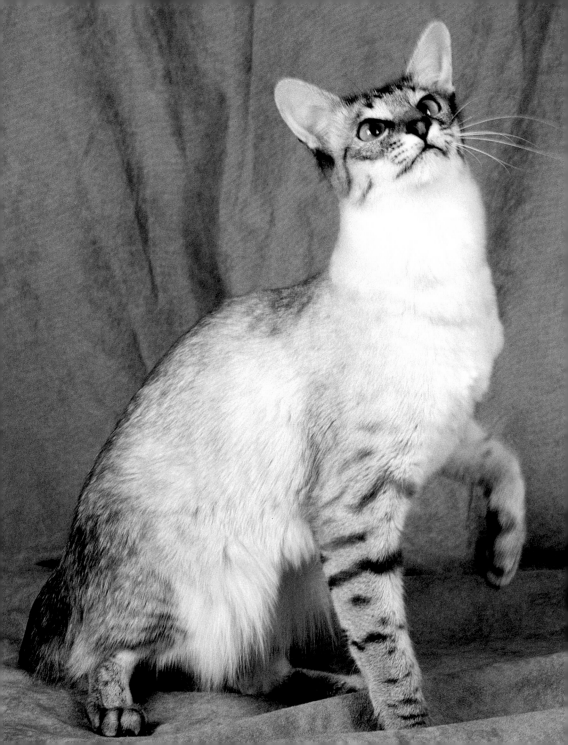

# JAVANESE

Quite similar in appearance and temperament to the Siamese and Balinese, this long-haired cat is only considered a separate breed because of its diversified coat color. It is also considered to be the long-haired version of the Colorpoint Shorthair; in fact, most Javanese are the offspring of Balinese who were bred with a Colorpoint Shorthair to produce a veritable rainbow of colors. Despite the beautiful long hair, the single-coated Javanese does not mat. This is not an excuse for you to be lazy, but if you don't brush her hair every day, I won't tell.

The Javanese breed standard, except for color, is identical to that of the Balinese. The name "Javanese" was chosen because the island of Java is next to the island of Bali. No one is disturbed by the fact that the Javanese cat does not comes from Java. After all, the Balinese cat does not come from Bali. The Siamese *does* come from Siam, however.

## History

Today, most Javanese cats can trace their ancestry back to two foundation queens: Alonale's Willo-the-Wisp (Canada) and Mishna M'Lady of Su-Bali (California).

Many cat registries do not accept the Javanese as a separate breed, because the only real difference is color. The CFA does, however. Most fanciers believe that the personality of each Javanese is linked to her color, with red and cream considered the most "laid back." Unlike the Balinese and Siamese, though, the Javanese has vivid green eyes.

Javanese are very easy to groom and sometimes are said to be "the lazy person's long-haired cat." Their coat is technically described as "medium long," which means about 2 or 3 inches (5.1-7.6 cm) long on the body and fuller on the tail to create the "plume." The advantage to allergy sufferers is that this cat has no undercoat. Single-coated breeds tend to have less hair (and thus fewer allergens) floating around.

**Did You Know?**

Although similar to the Balinese, the Javanese is considered a separate breed because of its diversified coat color.

## Appearance and Temperament

*Javanese cats are the offspring of Balinese who were bred with a Colorpoint Shorthair to produce a veritable rainbow of colors. This is a Blue Lynx.*

Many say that the Javanese is the Balinese "dipped in the colors of the rainbow." It is true that the only official difference in the breed standards is the color variations, but there must be magic in color, because the Javanese *seems* different. Perhaps it's because of all the difficulties breeders went through to get this cat recognized as a separate breed, but somehow the Javanese has the look and feel of an animal who has at least truly *arrived*, and her arrival has changed the cat scene forever.

The Cat Fanciers' Association claims that each color Javanese has a unique personality, although no real research shows this to be true. Like all cats, these are individuals who scorn typecasting. While most enjoy human companionship

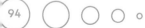

Javanese may appear fragile, but they are in fact quite muscular and capable of acrobatic feats and will delight you with their silly antics.

and will occasionally allow you to amuse yourself by watching them run after and destroy a toy, they may unaccountably "switch off," curl their swirl of a tail around that elegant head, and descend into the deep cat dreamland where no one can follow. The Javanese may pretend to miss you when you are gone and even become quite despondent. Don't believe it, though.

This is a breed for anyone who wants a little spice in their life. Although Javanese appear fragile, they are in fact quite muscular and capable of acrobatic feats. They are highly intelligent and quickly become familiar with your routine. They will often speak their minds to let you know what they need, whether it be a meal, some playtime, or just some attention. Considered a "busy" breed, these cats often seem to have nothing better to occupy their time than to follow you around and get underfoot. When they get tired of that, they spend a lot of time opening closets and unwrapping birthday presents. If you catch them at it, they will pretend they are hunting for mice, but it's all an act. They are much too elegant to chow down on flea-ridden rodents. Yet, they will delight in entertaining you with silly antics.

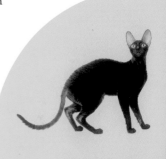

Javanese have colorful personalities. Their moods can range from playful and comical to aloof and sedate.

The Javanese has a notoriously fast metabolism, and so is in less danger than many other breeds of becoming overweight. Most of them can free-feed without losing their svelte, elegant shape. Their zest for play also helps burn off those extra calories.

Health problems in the breed include congenital heart defects, crossed eyes, and nystagmus, a rapid back-and-forth motion of the eyes that does not impair their vision. They may also suffer from

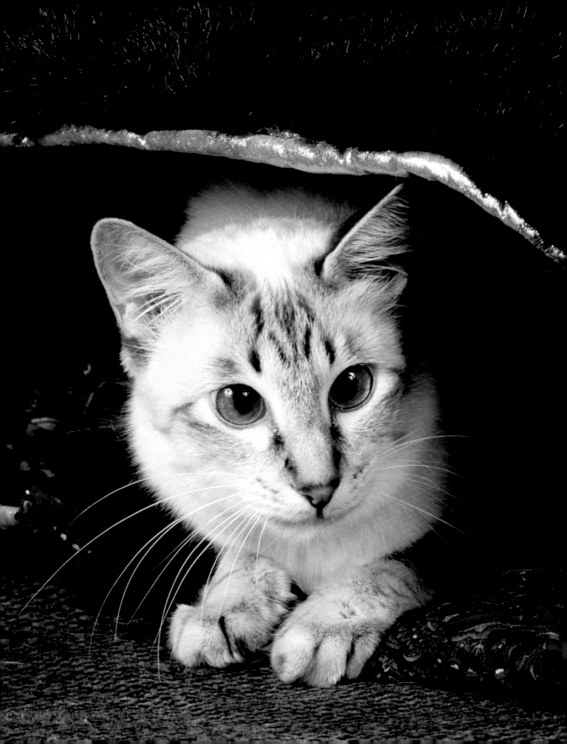

some of the same problems as Siamese, such as endocardial fibroelastosis and protrusion of the cranial sternum.

The Javanese may be outcrossed with the Balinese, Colorpoint Shorthair, and Siamese.

## Association Acceptance

The Javanese is accepted by the Cat Fanciers' Association (CFA).

---

# THE JAVANESE AT A GLANCE

**General Appearance:** Svelte, strong, tapering body. Appearance softened by the long coat.

**Head:** Long tapering wedge. Medium size. Skull flat, no bulge over the eyes or dip in the nose.

**Ears:** Very large, pointed, wide at the base.

**Eyes:** Almond shaped. Medium size. Slanted toward the nose.

**Neck:** Long and slender.

**Nose:** Long and straight.

**Muzzle:** Fine and wedge shaped.

**Chin and Jaw:** Medium size.

**Body:** Medium, graceful, long.

**Legs:** Long and slim.

**Paws:** Dainty and small, oval. Five toes in front, four in back.

**Tail:** Plumy.

**Coat::** Medium length, fine, silky.

**Colors:** Body colors must be even, with subtle shading when allowed. Mask, ears, legs, feet, and tail colors should be dense and clearly defined.

**Faults:** Lack of pigment in the nose leather or paw pads. Crossed eyes.

**Disqualifications:** Evidence of illness, weak hind legs. Malocclusion. Kink in the tail.

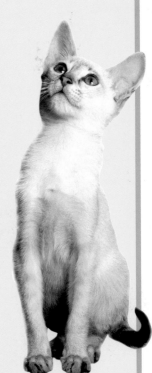

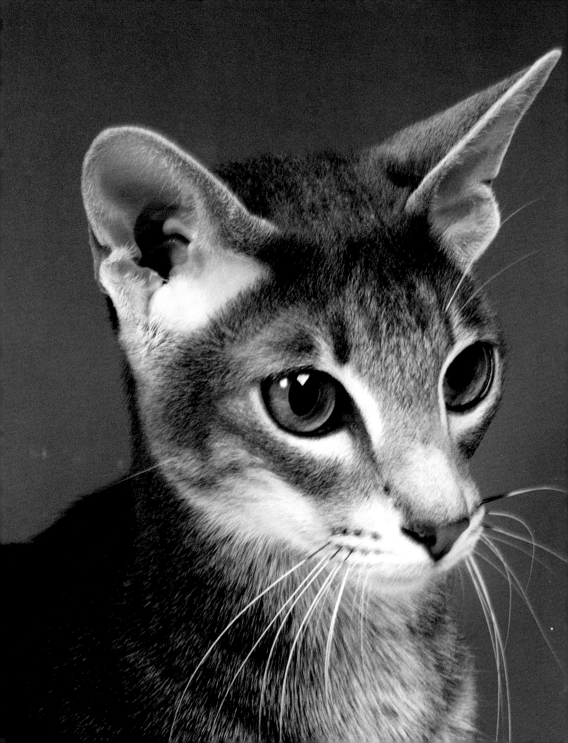

# ORIENTAL SHORTHAIR

The sleek and elegant Oriental Shorthair comes in more than 300 colors. The coat is silky and lies close to the body. This breed has the general physical characteristics of the Siamese.

These cats are playful well into their later years and affectionately greet their owners on sight, looking for the attention they so desperately crave. Spirited and loyal, their lively personalities make them fun to have around, but they are also equally comfortable snuggling up to you for some quiet time at the end of a long day.

## History

Let's go back in time to a very old manuscript called the *Cat-Book Poems*. Written in Thailand (which used to be Siam), there are descriptions and pictures of the cats we all recognize as Siamese. But there's something odd about some of them. Instead of the typical Siamese coloring, we see solid black cats, blue-gray cats, brown cats, and some shaded silver. In fact, cats of all these colors were regularly transported to England and elsewhere as Siamese. It was not until the 1920s, when the Siamese Cat Club simply banished from its registry all animals other than the blue-eyed, color-pointed cats that we recognize today as the Siamese that the distinction became necessary. Their unrecognized brethren faded away into the general cat population.

Today's version of the Oriental is not a direct import from Thailand but a hybrid developed in the 1950s and 1960s. It was deliberately created to

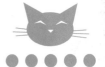

The Oriental Shorthair comes in more than 300 colors.

retain the Siamese body type and character but with different colors added. Domestic shorthairs, Russian Blues, and Abyssinians were called into service, with dutiful backcrossing performed regularly to keep the type pure. The breed was accepted in 1972 by the CFA for registration, with championship status coming in 1977. Since that time, the breed has steadily gained in popularity. There is a long-haired and short-haired version of this breed, with the shorter coat perhaps being more hypoallergenic.

## Appearance and Temperament

While the CFA breed profile claims that the Oriental "desperately" wishes to share her life with you, I wouldn't be too sure about this. She is quite happy for you to devote yourself to her care and keeping, and she will probably shower you with a good deal of attention—for a cat. But don't forget that the Oriental is always looking out for herself first. She wants you there, no doubt about it, but you'll be better received if you pay her all due attention.

The Oriental is as talky as the Siamese, but owners claim that her conversations are more sedate and possibly more logical. This cat definitely plays favorites, but you can worm yourself into her good graces with a few well-chosen bribes.

Even though Orientals are less allergy provoking than other breeds, it's still a good idea to get someone to brush the cat, which helps to reduce dander. The best brush to use on a short-haired coat is the solid rubber curry type. It should be placed in the palm of the hand with the curved side out; this side is designed to remove loose, dead, or extra hair. Brush thoroughly using long strokes in the direction that the hair grows. You can also run a damp cloth especially designed to remove allergens along the fur to gather up loose hairs.

Orientals are generally healthy, but because they are closely related to Siamese, they share some of the same diseases, notably gum disease, amyloidosis (a liver-destroying disease), and cardiomyopathy. Some lines are also prone to endocardial fibroelastosis (a disorder that causes thickening of the heart muscle), which is a serious problem.

Allowable outcrosses include Siamese or Colorpoint.

## Association Acceptance

The Oriental Shorthair is accepted by CFA as a division of the Oriental breed and in TICA as part of the Siamese/Balinese/Oriental

Talkative and energetic, the Oriental Shorthair is an outgoing, people-oriented breed.

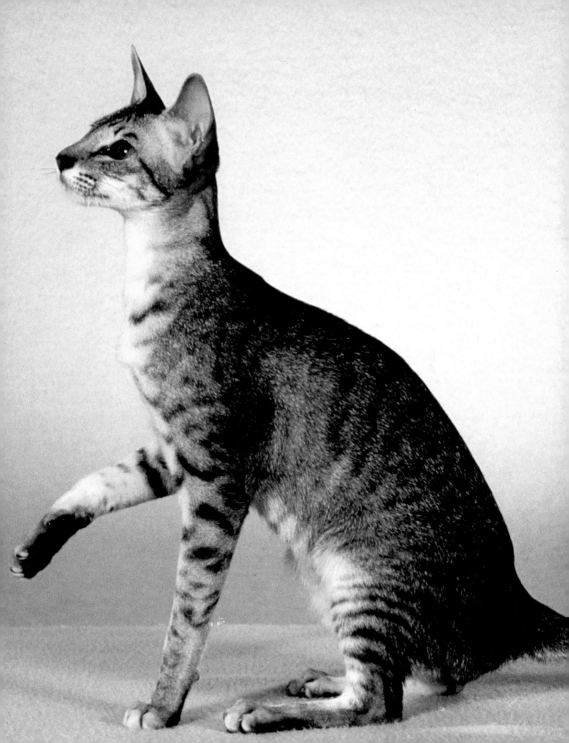

Shorthair/Oriental Longhair breed group. The AACE, ACA, ACFA, and UFO accept the Oriental Longhair as a breed in its own right.

- American Association of Cat Enthusiasts (AACE)
- American Cat Association (ACA)
- American Cat Fanciers Association (ACFA)
- Canadian Cat Association (CCA)
- Cat Fanciers' Association (CFA)
- Cat Fanciers Federation (CFF)
- The International Cat Association (TICA)
- United Feline Organization (UFO)

*Spirited and loyal, the Oriental's lively personality makes him fun to have around.*

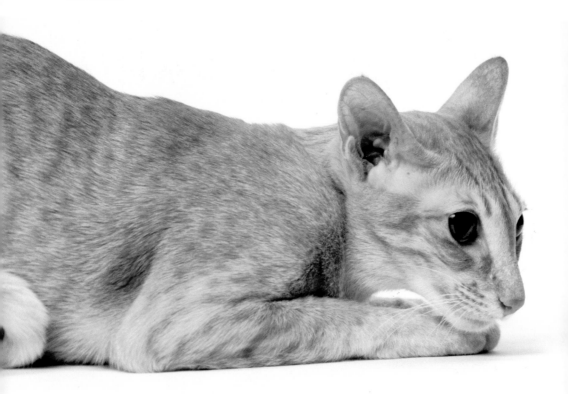

# THE ORIENTAL SHORTHAIR AT A GLANCE

**General Appearance:** Svelte and tubular. The breed comes in more than 300 allowable colors, including shaded, smoked, solid, bicolor, particolor, and tabby crosses. .

**Head:** Long tapering wedge. Flat skull.

**Nose:** Long and straight.

**Muzzle:** Fine, wedge shaped.

**Chin and Jaw:** Medium size. Tip of chin lines up with tip of nose in the same vertical plane.

**Ears:** Very large, pointed, and wide at the base.

**Eyes:** Almond shaped, medium size. Green. White Orientals and bicolor Orientals may have blue, green, or odd-eye color.

**Neck:** Long and slender.

**Body:** Long and svelte.

**Legs:** Long and slim, hind legs longer than front.

**Paws:** Dainty, small, and oval.

**Faults:** Crossed eyes. Palpable or visible protrusion of the cartilage at the end of the sternum.

**Disqualifications:** Any evidence of illness or poor health. Weak hind legs, emaciation, visible kinks in the tail.

## RESOURCES

### Registry Organizations

**American Association of Cat Enthusiasts (AACE)**
P.O. Box 213
Pine Brook, NJ 07058
Phone: (973) 335-6717
Website: http://www.aaceinc.org

**American Cat Fanciers Association (ACFA)**
P.O. Box 1949
Nixa, MO 65714
Phone: (417) 725-1530
Website: http://www.acfacat.com

**Canadian Cat Association (CCA)**
289 Rutherford Road South
Unit 18
Brampton, Ontario, Canada L6W 3R9
Phone: (905) 459-1481
Website: http://www.cca-afc.com

**The Cat Fanciers' Association (CFA)**
1805 Atlantic Avenue
P.O. Box 1005
Manasquan, NJ 08736-0805
Phone: (732) 528-9797
Website: http://www.cfainc.org

**Cat Fanciers' Federation (CFF)**
P.O. Box 661
Gratis, OH 45330
Phone: (937) 787-9009
Website: http://www.cffinc.org

**Fédération Internationale Féline (FIFe)**
Penelope Bydlinski, General Secretary
Little Dene, Lenham Heath
Maidstone, Kent, ME17 2BS ENGLAND
Phone: +44 1622 850913
Website: http://www.fifeweb.org

**The Governing Council of the Cat Fancy (GCCF)**
4-6, Penel Orlieu
Bridgwater, Somerset, TA6 3PG UK
Phone: +44 (0)1278 427 575
Website:
http://ourworld.compuserve.com/homepages/GCCF_CATS/

**The International Cat Association (TICA)**
P.O. Box 2684
Harlingen, TX 78551
Phone: (956) 428-8046
Website: http://www.tica.org

**Traditional and Classic Cat International (TCCI)**
(formerly known as the Traditional Cat Association)
10289 Vista Point Loop
Penn Valley, CA 95946
Website: http://www.tccat.org

### Websites

**Acme Pet Feline Guide**
(http://www.acmepet.com/feline/index.html)
A leading figure in the pet products industry, Acme Pet has put together an extensive site. At the feline site, you can access the feline marketplace, which has places to shop for cat products as well as a pet library, reference materials and articles, questions and answers about cats, an extensive list of rescue organizations, clubs and shelters, and the ever popular "cat chat" room.

**Cat Collectors**
(http://www.catcollectors.com)
This club is designed for people who collect cat-related items (such as figurines, books, artwork, advertisements, and other items that bear a cat motif), and is the first of its kind. Club founder, Marilyn Dipboye, started Cat Collectors in 1982 so that the people who enjoy this hobby can network with each other, whether selling or

trading certain pieces or just sharing friendships. A newsletter, Cat Talk, is mailed bi-monthly to its members.

## Cat Fanciers Website
(http://www.fanciers.com)
In 1993, the Cat Fanciers mailing list was started on the Internet as an open forum for breeders, exhibitors, judges, or anyone interested in the world of the Cat Fancy. The on-line discussion group has thousands of members from all over the world. The group's focus, however, is to make life better for felines around the globe. The site offers general information on cat
shows, breed descriptions, veterinary resources, and much more.

## The Daily Cat
(http://www.thedailycat.com)
The Daily Cat is a resource for cats and their owners. The site provides information on feline health, care, nutrition, grooming, and behavior.

## Healthypet
(http://www.healthypet.com)
Healthypet.com is part of the American Animal Hospital Association, an organization of more than 25,000 veterinary care providers committed to providing excellence in small animal care.

## Petfinder
(http://www.petfinder.org)
On Petfinder.org, you can search over 88,000 adoptable animals and locate shelters and rescue groups in your area who are currently caring for adoptable pets. You can also post classified ads for lost or found pets, pets wanted, and pets needing homes.

## Pets 911
(http://www.1888pets911.org)
Pets 911 is not only a website, but also runs a toll-free phone hotline (1-888-PETS-911) that allows pet owners access to important, life-saving information.

## ShowCatsOnline
(http://www.showcatsonline.com)
ShowCatsOnline.com is an online magazine devoted
to all breeds of pedigreed cats. They provide informa-tion on the breeding and showing of all breeds of
pedigreed cats and update their members on the latest developments in medical care, breeding, grooming,
and showing.

## 21cats.org
(http://21cats.org)
21Cats provides information that will help cats live longer, healthier lives. The site contains online Health and Care InfoCenter, an 'Ask the Kitty Nurse' Hotline, and a free monthly newsletter. One of their goals is to raise awareness of successful methods used to reduce the cat overpopulation problem.

## VetQuest
(http://www.vin.com/vetquest/index0.html)
VetQuest is an online veterinary search and referral service. You can search their database for over 25,000 Veterinary Hospitals and Clinics in the United States, Canada, and Europe. The service places special emphasis on veterinarians with advanced online access to the latest health care information and highly qualified veterinary specialists and consultants.

Publications

*Animal Wellness Magazine*
PMB 168
8174 South Holly Street
Centennial, CO 80122

*ASPCA Animal Watch*
424 East 92nd Street
New York, NY 10128

*Best Friends Magazine*
Best Friends Animal Sanctuary
Kanab, UT 84741

*Cat Fancy Magazine*
P.O. Box 52864
Boulder, CO 80322

*Catnip*
P.O. Box 420070
Palm Coast, FL 32142

*CatWatch*
P.O. Box 420235
Palm Coast, FL 32142

*PetLife Magazine*
P.O. Box 500
Missouri, TX 77549

*Whole Cat Journal*
P.O. Box 1337
Radford, VA 24143

*Your Cat Magazine*
1716 Locust Street
Des Moines, IA 50309

Veterinarian Specialty/Membership
Organizations

**American Animal Hospital Association
(AAHA)**
P.O. Box 150899
Denver, CO 80215
Phone: (303) 986-2800
Website: http://www.aahanet.org

**American Association of Feline Practitioners
(AAFP)**
200 4th Avenue North, Suite 900
Nashville, TN 37219
Phone: (615) 259-7788
Toll-free: (800) 204-3514
Website: http://www.aafponline.org

**American Board of Veterinary Practitioners
(ABVP)**
200 4th Avenue North, Suite 900
Nashville, TN 37219
Phone: (615) 254-3687
Fax: (615) 254-7047
Website: http://www.abvp.com

**American College of Veterinary Preventive
Medicine (ACVPM)**
3126 Morning Creek
San Antonio, TX 78247
Website: http://www.acvpm.org

**American Holistic Veterinary Medical
Association (AHVMA)**
2214 Old Emmorton Road
Bel Air, MD 21015
Phone: (410) 569-0795
Website: http://www.ahvma.org

**American Veterinary Medical Association
(AVMA)**
1931 North Meacham Road, Suite 100
Schaumburg, IL 60173
Phone: (847) 925-8070
Fax: (847) 925-1329
Website: http://www.avma.org

**The Academy of Veterinary Homeopathy
(AVH)**
P.O. Box 9280
Wilmington, DE 19809
Phone: (866) 652-1590
Website: http://www.theavh.org

**The American Association for Veterinary Acupuncture (AAVA)**
P.O. Box 419
Hygiene, CO 80533
Phone: (303) 772-6726
Website: http://www.aava.org

**Cornell Feline Health Center**
College of Veterinary Medicine
Cornell University, Box 13
Ithaca, NY 14853
Phone: (607) 253-3414
Website:
http://web.vet.cornell.edu/public/fhc/FelineHealth
.html

**International Veterinary Acupuncture Society (IVAS)**
P.O. Box 271395
Ft. Collins, CO 80527
Phone: (970) 266-0666
Website: http://www.ivas.org

Animal Welfare Groups and Organizations

**Alley Cat Allies**
1801 Belmont Road NW, Suite 201
Washington, DC 20009
Phone: (202) 667-3630
Website: http://www.alleycat.org

**American Humane Association (AHA)**
63 Inverness Drive East
Englewood, CO 80112
Phone: (800) 227-4645
Website: http://www.americanhumane.org

**American Society for the Prevention of Cruelty**
to Animals (ASPCA)
424 East 92 Street
New York, NY 10128
Phone: (212) 876-7700
Website: http://www.aspca.org

**Best Friends Animal Sanctuary**
Kanab, UT 84741-5001
Phone: (435) 644-2001
Website: http://www.bestfriends.org

**Cats Protection**
17 Kings Road
Horsham, West Sussex RH13 5PN UK
Phone: +44 (0) 1403 221900
Website: http://www.cats.org.uk

**Feral Cat Coalition**
9528 Miramar Road, PMB 160
San Diego, CA 92126
Phone: (619) 497-1599
Website: http://www.feralcat.com

**The Fund For Animals**
200 West 57th Street
New York, NY 10019
Phone: (212) 246-2096
Website: http://www.fund.org

**The Humane Society of the United States (HSUS)**
2100 L Street, NW
Washington, DC 20037
Phone: (212) 452-1100
Website: http://www.hsus.org

**North Shore Animal League (NSAL)**
25 Davis Avenue
Port Washington, NY 11050
Phone: (516) 883-7575
Website: http://www.nsal.org

**The Winn Feline Foundation, Inc.**
1805 Atlantic Avenue
P.O. Box 1005
Manasquan, NJ 08736-0805
Phone: (732) 528-9797
Website: http://www.winnfelinehealth.org

# INDEX

*Note: Boldface indicates illustrations*

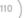

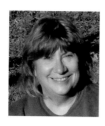

## About the Author

Diane Morgan is an award-winning writer who is the author of many books on pet care, including *Sneeze-Free Dog Breeds*, *Good Dogkeeping*, *The Quick and Easy Guide to Bird Care*, and *Feeding Your Horse for Life*. She is a college professor of philosophy and literature and resides in Williamsport, Maryland with seven dogs, two humans, and an uncounted number of goldfish.

## Acknowledgments

To my many friends at Cumberland Valley Veterinary Clinic. You guys are the very best!
Also, grateful thanks to Mary Grangeia, super editor, who really turned this manuscript into a book.

## Photo Credits

Linda Beatie: 101; Anne Gro Bergersen (Shutterstock): 76; Pam Burley (Shutterstock): 13, 25; Alex James Bramwell (Shutterstock): 39; Natalia Bratslavsky (Shutterstock): 46; Stephen Coburn (Shutterstock): 44; Lawrence Cruciana (Shutterstock): 7; S. Duffet (Shutterstock): 47; Jaimie Duplass (Shutterstock): 26; Isabelle Francais: 1, 3, 23, 53, 54, 55, 59, 60, 62, 64, 66, 67, 68, 69, 70, 72, 74, 75, 78, 79, 83, 85, 86, 87, 90, 91, 92, 94, 96, 99, 102, 103; Keith A. Frith (Shutterstock): 28; Gajatz (Shutterstock): 36; Eric Gevaert (Shutterstock): 49; Johanna Goodyear (Shutterstock): 51; Ken Hurst (Shutterstock): 30; Indigo Fish (Shutterstock): 58; Vadim Kozlovsky (Shutterstock): 17; Anthony Mahadevan (Shutterstock): 4; Suponev Vladimir Mihajlovich (Shutterstock): 41; Michelle D. Milliman (Shutterstock): 8; Jeff Oien (Shutterstock): 10 ; Ruben Paz (Shutterstock): 34; Michael Pettigrew (Shutterstock): 9; Elena Ray (Shutterstock): 32; Ron Regan: 80; Spauln (Shutterstock): 20; Tatiana (Shutterstock): 57; Tiburon Studios (Shutterstock): 18; Troy (Shutterstock): 15; Graca Victoria (Shutterstock): 12; Mayer George Vladimirovich (Shutterstock): 42; Front and cover photos: Isabelle Francais, TFH Archives